"As an indication of the educational importance and practical relevance of Dr. Chaney's new book, I read every word of every page. **Slaying the Supplement Myths** presents an amazing amount of information on food supplements, with evidence-based guidelines for separating fact from fiction. Dr. Chaney is a highly-respected researcher who has exceptional breadth of knowledge and depth of understanding as related to nutrition and health. He has the admirable ability to identify studies with confounding factors, and studies that are conducted carefully, comprehensively, and correctly, with appropriate conclusions and applications. I learned far more than I anticipated from this extremely well-researched and well-written book, even with very high expectations before I began reading. If you want to make the best supplement decisions based on the best research studies, this is the book that will enable you to do so."

Dr. Wayne Westcott, Professor of Exercise Science at Quincy College and Fitness Research Director at the South Shore YMCA in Quincy, MA. Dr. Westcott is the author of 20 fitness books and has been honored with the Lifetime Achievement Award from the International Association on Fitness Professionals.

"This book eliminates much of the confusion that many customers have about the dietary supplement industry. It is well-written and packed with content that is informative, yet captivating. The common myths are dispelled, and Dr. Chaney concludes with practical tips for choosing the right dietary supplements."

David A. Colby, Pharm.D., Ph.D.
Associate Professor of Medicinal Chemistry and Research Associate Professor in the Research Institute of Pharmaceutical Sciences
University of Mississippi School of Pharmacy

"It's all too easy to get confused by the media hype, trends, science and "psuedo" science that surrounds supplementation and changes every few months. Who can you trust and what should you believe? In his latest book "Slaying the Supplement Myths", Dr Stephen Chaney breaks down the last 30 years of myths and confusion to empower the reader with everything needed to know and evaluate good nutrition and supplementation decisions for your health. What's good? What's bad? Will soy give you cancer? Can fruits and vegetables really be put in a capsule? Is enhanced water really good for you? What's junk science and what's real? How can you chart a course that's best for the health of you and your family... and be confident the science won't change in a few months? Dr Chaney is seasoned veteran scientist who answers all those questions and more. If you're looking for the real deal, then grab a copy of this book, read it, and share it with your friends and family. The knowledge and advice that Dr Chaney covers in these pages is essential for everyone who wants the best for their health."

Sean Greeley, CEO, NPE, 8 times Inc 500/5000 Global
Fitness Business Coaching Company

SLAYING THE SUPPLEMENT MYTHS

THE TRUTH BEHIND THE HYPE

DR. STEVE CHANEY, PhD

Paperback ISBN: 978-1-64184-951-7

Ebook ISBN: 978-1-64184-952-4

Book design by JETLAUNCH.net

About The Author

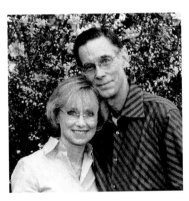 Dr. Steve Chaney received his B.S. degree in Chemistry from Duke University and his Ph.D. degree in Biochemistry from UCLA. He is currently Professor Emeritus at the University of North Carolina at Chapel Hill. At the time of his retirement he held the title of Distinguished Professor in the Department of Biochemistry and Biophysics and the Department of Nutrition.

Dr. Chaney is:

- A bestselling author. His recent book "Slaying The Food Myths" was an Amazon best seller in 3 categories.

- An award-winning educator who taught human metabolism and nutrition to first year medical and dental students for 40 years. He was named "Basic Science Teacher of the Year" several times by the first-year medical students and was awarded the "Excellence in Teaching Lifetime Achievement Award" by the Academy of Educators upon his retirement in 2012.

- An internationally recognized scientist who ran an active cancer research program for 37 years. He has published over 100 papers and 12 reviews in peer-reviewed scientific journals. He helped develop a drug that represents a major advance in the treatment of colon cancer and was a featured speaker at 6 international symposia on anticancer drugs.

- A recognized nutrition expert who was asked to write two chapters on nutrition for the first 6 editions of "Textbook of Biochemistry With Clinical Correlations", one of the leading biochemistry textbooks for medical students.

- A sought-after speaker on creating healthier lifestyles.

Upon his retirement from the University of North Carolina Dr. Chaney founded his "Health Tips From The Professor" (https://healthtipsfromtheprofessor.com) weekly blog. His mission is to cut through the hype and myths to provide you with the truth about how you can attain and maintain optimal health. He takes the headlines of the day, analyzes the research behind them, and tells you whether you should trust them or ignore them.

In his 40 years of teaching medical students and public speaking, Dr. Chaney realized just how confusing supplementation was to the average person. One day, supplements are going to cure you. The next day they are going to kill you. One day, fish oil is good for you. The next day it is called snake oil. Dr. Chaney has searched the literature to find science-based information on supplementation. He will guide you through the maze of claims and counter claims, so you can choose a supplement program that is best for you.

On the other hand, there are supplement companies with no quality controls and no proof their products work. There are companies that lie to you, and companies that manufacture products they know are dangerous. In this book Dr. Chaney shines a light into the dark corners of the supplement industry. He guides you through the maze of incompetence, lies, and deception so you can choose supplements that are both safe and effective.

Foreword

Considering my early years, I might be considered the least likely person to be writing a book about nutrition and health, particularly one that features the lies and myths about supplementation.

Growing up, I ate a typical American diet. As a teenager, my favorite places to eat were Amado's Pizza and the Charburger Grill (the name says it all). In my 20s, I never thought much about nutrition, or that what I ate could affect my health. I never thought about supplementation. After all, my mother had taught me that my "balanced diet" would provide everything I needed. As a college student, I often got colds. I was usually tired by mid-afternoon. I thought that was normal. After all, I was a typical student. I kept crazy hours. I just needed an over-the-counter cold medicine and more coffee.

In graduate school my life started to change. I met my beautiful and amazing soulmate, Suzanne. She had been raised by a mom who believed in natural, holistic approaches to health – including a healthy diet and supplementation. By the standards of her time, her mom was a "health nut." Actually, she was way ahead of her time.

When Suzanne and I got married, her cooking was very different from what I was used to. I was eating healthier, but I never thought about it. It was not a conscious decision on my part. Encouraged by my mother-in-law, I began to investigate the impact of diet on health outcomes. My mother-in-law encouraged me to read various health magazines in addition to the scientific literature I was reading for my graduate studies. Of course, I didn't automatically believe everything I read in those magazines. As a graduate student, I was a "skeptic in training." I checked out what those magazines had to say by reading the pertinent scientific literature. I rejected a lot of what I read, but some of it rang true. Little by little I learned how important good nutrition and a healthy lifestyle were to my overall health. More importantly, I learned how to separate fact from fiction.

The changes in diet and lifestyle that I have made over the years have paid off. I am now in my 70s and am in perfect health, with no illnesses and no medications. As I look back, I wish I could have told my younger self what I know now. More importantly, I wanted to share that information with so many young people who, like my earlier self, know nothing about nutrition and how important it is to their health. I wanted these young people to enjoy the same health when they reach their golden years as I enjoy today. I also realized how hard it was for the average person to sort through the myths about healthy foods and diet that abound in today's world. I wanted to give people a guide, so they could cut through the misinformation and discover the truth about healthy eating. That was the genesis of my first book, which I called "**Slaying the Food Myths**."

In addition to cooking nutritious meals, my wife put a multivitamin by my plate every day. I didn't think much about it. I just considered it part of the meal and took it. I started to feel better. I had more energy. I had fewer colds. That roused my curiosity. Could that multivitamin actually have made a difference? Remember, I was a "skeptic in training." I knew about the placebo effect. I started scanning the scientific literature, so I could also separate fact from fiction about supplementation. I learned that, under the appropriate conditions, supplementation was effective. I also learned that there was a lot of hype and misinformation about supplementation. Again, I realized how hard it is for people to sort through the supplement myths. That was the genesis of this book, which I call **"Slaying the Supplement Myths."**

As I was learning about supplementation, my mother-in-law was telling me about the quality of the supplements she was using. I was impressed, but not convinced at first. I assumed that the FDA regulated the supplement industry in the same way it regulated the drug industry. As I learned more, I was horrified to find out that was not the case. Quality controls were not required in those days. While a few companies were making high quality supplements, many companies were not. They had no quality controls. You had no idea what you were getting. Their products might have little or no active ingredients. They might have impurities. They might even have dangerous contaminants.

My mother-in-law also talked about the clinical proof behind the supplements she was using. Again, I had assumed that the FDA must surely require supplement manufacturers to conduct clinical studies proving that their products were safe and effective. Once again, I was sorely disappointed. The FDA did not require proof of safety and efficacy in the supplement industry.

When you think about it, this is the worst of all possible worlds. There are supplements on the market with no quality controls and no proof that they work. Yet if you look at their literature, it sounds like these supplements are as pure as the driven snow and can cure all your ills. What I have learned about the dark side of the food supplement industry over the years is the basis for the section in this book titled "**The Lies of the Charlatans.**"

Like everyone else, I was also confused by all the conflicting headlines about supplementation in my younger years. One day you were told nutrient "X" would cure you. The next day you were told it would kill you. Over my 40 years of scientific research I had become quite skilled at analyzing the strengths and weaknesses of scientific publications. Eventually, I started to use these skills to analyze the publications behind the headlines, so I could determine which of them were bogus and which were true. The more I learned, the more I wanted to share this information with others. I knew the conflicting headlines must be just as confusing to others as they had been for me.

However, most people simply don't have the scientific background to separate fact from fiction. I wanted to help others cut through the misleading headlines and nutrition myths. I wanted to tell them which headlines to ignore and which to trust. The misleading information on the benefits of supplementation made its way into "The Lies of the Charlatans" section. The misleading information on the dangers of supplementation formed the basis for the section in this book titled "**The Myths of the Naysayers.**"

Dr. Steve Chaney, PhD

P.S. In addition to this book I have created a weekly blog called "Health Tips From the Professor" (https://healthtipsfromtheprofessor.com). Each week I start with a recent headline, analyze the study behind the headline, and give a balanced, scientifically sound evaluation of the claim(s) made in the headline. I tell you whether you should ignore the headline or act on it. In addition, I have started providing educational Facebook Live videos on my Steve Chaney Facebook page.

Acknowledgements

I would like to start by acknowledging my beautiful wife Suzanne who has put up with a skeptical professor and kept him healthy all these years. They say that "Behind every successful man there is a good woman." I would reword that to say: "Behind every healthy man there is a wise woman." However, Suzanne is much more than that. She is my companion and soulmate. She is also very successful in her own right.

I would like to acknowledge my mother-in-law, Mary Becker, who was my inspiration and my guide. I would like to acknowledge my son Marc, who encouraged me to write this book. Finally, I would like to acknowledge my daughter-in-law, Ashley. Marc and Ashley already know much more about nutrition than I did at their age and are raising our granddaughter, Kaziah Grace, with love and good nutrition.

Disclaimer

The statements in this book have not been approved by the Food and Drug Administration. They are not intended to diagnose, treat, cure, or prevent disease. More importantly, the information in the book is not meant to replace the advice of your health professional. Rather, it is meant to be something you discuss with your health professional as you partner together to create your healthy living plan.

Table Of Contents

Section 1: The Lies Of The Charlatans

Section 2: The Myths of the Naysayers

SLAYING THE SUPPLEMENT MYTHS

Section 1: The Lies Of The Charlatans

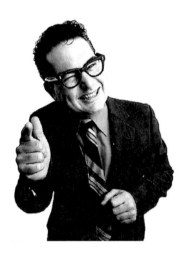

Did you know that some supplement companies…

   …manufacture products that are worthless or contaminated?

      …have no proof their products are either safe or effective?

         …manufacture products they know are dangerous?

         …lie to you?

   I have shined a light into the dark corners of the supplement industry

I will guide you through the maze of hype, incompetence, lies, and deception, so you can choose supplements that are both safe and effective.

Overview

In my first book, "Slaying the Food Myths," I summarized the reasons why a common-sense supplementation program is a valuable addition to a healthy diet. In fact, I believe supplementation should be an integral component of anyone's holistic program for a healthier lifestyle. However, I don't need to tell you that supplementation is controversial.

That's because the world of supplementation is full of charlatans, liars and naysayers. There are a lot of people telling you what you should be thinking about supplementation. You know that all the things you are hearing can't be true. So, you are probably asking yourself what is the truth about supplementation? My message to you is to question what you've been told, or, put another way, rethink what you have come to believe.

On the one hand, you're being told about supplements that will make the pounds melt away effortlessly. They're going to make you live to 150. They're going to cure what ails you. Some of the stories even seem to suggest that they're going to heal the lame and raise the dead. I'm exaggerating a little bit, but if you read some of the hype out there, it almost sounds that good.

The problem is that the websites and sales people sound so convincing. They start with intriguing stories about how this food or herb is only known to monks in the high Himalayas... or to some South Pacific islanders...or to natives in the deepest Amazon jungle – just to give a few examples. Their stories often say that their amazing product is based on the research of a dedicated scientist, but that it is being suppressed by the pharmaceutical industry and/or the medical profession because it would put them out of business.

Then they add testimonials that are dramatic and compelling – people telling amazing stories about how this product has transformed their lives. It's tempting to think, "If so many other people are getting fantastic results, maybe I should give it a try."

What you don't realize is that many of these testimonials are "made up." The company has simply downloaded some photos from the internet and made up stories to go with them. Even when the testimonials do come from real people, you need to know about something called "the placebo effect".

The word placebo comes from the Latin and means "I shall please". The original definition of placebo was "a measure designed to calm or please someone rather than to provide any real benefit". The term placebo entered the medical realm in recognition of the fact that the mere act of a doctor or an expert recommending a pill or treatment had a psychological benefit for a patient. In this context, a placebo is defined as "a harmless pill, medicine, or treatment prescribed more for the psychological benefit to the patient than for any physiological effect".

In short, our minds are powerful. If we believe strongly enough that a pill or treatment will make us feel better, we can actually experience a feeling of well-being that has no basis in reality. That psychological feeling of well-being is what we refer to as "the placebo effect". For things like pain relief, energy and feelings of well-being the placebo effect approaches 50%. That is why you always need to be skeptical about testimonials unless they are backed by clinical trials showing the product works. That is why the best clinical trials include a control group that receives a placebo.

You also should know that as little as 10 pounds of weight loss will lower cholesterol levels, improve blood sugar control, and lower blood pressure. Many of the reported health benefits for their product may have simply come from a change in diet or a bit of weight loss and have nothing to do with all the fancy ingredients in the supplement.

Finally, many of these companies will give you a long list of endorsements by doctors, athletes, and other famous people attesting to the value of their product. What you need to know is that endorsements are commodities. They are bought and sold.

My advice is to ignore the intriguing stories, the compelling testimonials, and the endorsements and focus on products that are backed by solid science. Unfortunately, even that is not easy. Many companies try to dazzle you with what I call junk science rather than real science (I will tell you how to distinguish between junk science and real science later in this section). Always remember that famous saying: "If it sounds too good to be true, it probably is [too good to be true]."

On the other hand, you're being told that vitamins don't work. They might cause cancer. They might give you heart attacks. They may even kill you. So, what are you to believe? Where is that truth?

That's why I wrote this book, which I call "Slaying the Supplement Myths." I have divided this book into two sections. In this section of the book, "The Lies of the Charlatans," I talk about the hype and misleading information about those "magic" supplements that promise to cure what ails you. I will also give you some practical guidelines on how to separate the hype from the facts.

In section 2, "The Myths of the Naysayers," I will talk about the negative hype – the naysayers and the "urban myths" about supplementation. I will also give you some practical guidelines on what a science-based supplementation program looks like and how to choose supplements you can trust.

1

The Lies of the Food Supplement Industry

Let's start by exposing some of the lies of the food supplement industry. (They may call it marketing. I call it lying.) I can't possibly cover all the lies, so I will just give you a few examples. If you pay attention, however, you will notice a common thread running through each of these examples. That thread is – If you really think about it, each of these claims sounds just a little too good to be true.

Fruits and Vegetables in a Capsule Con

In my first book, "Slaying The Food Myths," I told you about food manufacturers who sprinkle a little fruit and vegetable powder into their processed foods and try to fool you into thinking those foods are chock full of real fruits and vegetables.

Unfortunately, the same thing happens in the supplement industry. One of my pet peeves is the food supplement manufacturers who try to tell you that they have concentrated a cornucopia of fresh fruits and vegetables in a capsule.

For example, one company claims that their capsules contain apple, barley, broccoli, beet, cabbage, carrot, cranberry, date, garlic, kale, oats, orange, parsley, peach, pineapple, prunes, spinach, plant enzymes, fiber, and acidophilus. All this in one capsule!

While this list sounds impressive, you need to ask whether they are providing meaningful amounts of those fruits and vegetables. For example, the product claims to have oats. A serving of oats is equal to 1/3 cup dry oats and weighs about 28 grams. A capsule typically weighs about 0.5 grams. Therefore, to get the equivalent of one serving of oats from a capsule, you would have to consume 56 capsules! And that's assuming the entire capsule was filled with oats.

Broccoli is another claimed ingredient. A serving of fresh broccoli weighs 88 grams, but roughly 80 grams of that is water. So, if you dehydrated the broccoli, you would be left with about 8 grams of material. Therefore, to get a single serving of dehydrated broccoli you would have to consume 16 capsules. Again, that's assuming the capsules were completely filled with just broccoli.

You can do this kind of calculation with each ingredient they claim is in their capsules. But when you add up the number of capsules needed to get a reasonable amount of each of these ingredients, the capsule total is staggering.

As for essential nutrients, when you read the **Supplement Facts** portion of the label (that's the portion of the label that is required by the FDA) you often discover that the capsules only contain small amounts of a few essential nutrients. If they do list significant levels of micronutrients, that generally means that those micronutrients have been added to the supplement. Those micronutrients didn't come from the fruit and vegetable powders, and they are generally synthetic.

For example, I have seen supplements that claim they are all natural, with all their ingredients coming from fruits and vegetables. But, when you read the label, it lists ingredients that never saw a fruit or vegetable.

The bottom line is that the "whole foods" (which are actually fruit and vegetable powders purchased from their favorite supplier) that the manufacturers claim to have crammed into their supplements simply do not provide significant amounts of the vitamins and minerals you would have been getting if you ate the real foods.

"What about *phytonutrients*?", you might ask. Some manufacturers also claim that because they use "whole food" ingredients, their supplements are chock full of phytonutrients. Surely their supplements must be healthier than the other products in the marketplace. Not really!

Recently, a group of scientists[1] decided to test the claims of one of the companies who claim to make "whole food" supplements. They compared the nutrients obtained from eating broccoli sprouts and from eating a broccoli sprout pill. Yes, there are actually supplement manufacturers who market broccoli sprout pills. After all, everyone knows that broccoli is good for us, but many people don't like the taste of broccoli.

Before I describe the study, let me give you some background (I apologize in advance for the big words). One of the reasons that broccoli and other cruciferous vegetables are so healthy is that they contain sulfur-containing compounds called glucosinolates. Glucosinolates are relative inert by themselves, but they are converted by an enzyme called myrosinase to a class of compounds called *isothiocyanates*. Isothiocyanates are responsible for most of the health benefits of cruciferous vegetables, but they are very unstable. They are rapidly metabolized by the liver and excreted in the urine. For this reason, myrosinase is physically separated from the glucosinolates in the intact cell.

When we put a piece of raw broccoli or a broccoli sprout into our mouth and start chewing it, the myroinase is released and the glucosinolates are converted in to isothiocyanates. The isothiocyanates are rapidly absorbed into our blood-stream, where they can exert their beneficial effects before they are degraded and eliminated.

The major glucosinolate in broccoli sprouts is glucoraph-anin, and two of the major beneficial isothiocyanates derived from glucoraphanin are sulforaphane and erucic acid. Broccoli sprouts are ideally suited for providing you with high levels of sulforaphane and erucic acid because they contain both glucoraphanin and myrosinase. However, the story is more complicated for broccoli sprout supplements. It is easy to extract the glucoraphanin from broccoli, but it is much more difficult to extract and preserve the activity of myrosinase. Did the broccoli sprout supplements in this study contain myrosinase? Let's see.

The scientists started by giving the subjects 40 grams of fresh broccoli sprouts. Over the next 48 hours they measured the levels of sulforaphane and erucic acid in their blood and urine. After a one-month washout period, the same subjects took 6 broccoli sprout pills (which the manufacturer claimed were equivalent to 40 grams of broccoli sprouts) and the scien-tists again measured levels of the same beneficial nutrients in their blood and urine. The results were dramatic. The subjects had 4.5- to 7.4-fold higher levels of sulforaphane and erucic acid in their bloodstream and urine following consumption of broccoli sprouts than they did after taking broccoli sprout pills.

The story is similar with garlic supplements. In this case, the inert precursor is called alliin, the enzyme is called alliinase, and the biologically active derivative is called allicin. Allicin is also responsible for the odor associated with garlic. When you crush or chop a clove of garlic, alliinase is released and alliin is converted to allicin, creating both the smell and the health benefits of garlic. Once again, garlic supplements are a differ-ent story. Customers want the health benefits of garlic without the odor. The easiest way to make a garlic supplement odorless is to retain the alliin and remove the alliinase. Need I say more?

The Bottom Line: Leave those supplements claiming to have concentrated lots of fruits and vegetables into a single capsule on the shelf. Those claims are grossly deceptive because the capsules do not contain significant amounts of the fruits and vegetables listed on the label. They do not provide the nutrients and phytonutrients you would have gotten if you had eaten the real foods. Once again, the best way to get the fruits and vegetables you need in your diet is to actually eat fresh fruits and vegetables.

Final Word: Many of you have asked me about companies that claim their supplement has the amount of vitamin C found in 7 oranges or the amount of folic acid found in 4 cups of cooked green peas. Those are FDA-allowed claims and are generally accurate. Just don't assume that the vitamin C actually came from 7 oranges (it didn't) or that their supplement has all the nutrients found in 7 oranges (it doesn't).

"All Natural" Nonsense

Another deceptive marketing message is the "all natural" claim. These companies do not claim that they have squeezed a cornucopia of fresh fruits and vegetables into a tiny capsule, but they do claim, or imply, that their micronutrients were all derived from fresh fruits and vegetables. This is an equally outrageous claim.

Let's take folic acid, for example. The RDA for folic acid is 400 micrograms, so each capsule or tablet of most multivitamins and B complex supplements provides at least this much. If we look at the best food sources of folates and ask how much you would need to start with to end up with 400 micrograms of folic acid, the numbers are pretty astonishing.

It would take 1 cup of lentils, 2 cups of cooked spinach, 4 cups of cooked broccoli, 4 papayas or 10 cups of almonds to end up with 400 micrograms of folic acid. That's assuming 100% efficiency of extraction (which is impossible) and that all the folates in these foods were in the form of folic acid (they aren't). You also need to keep in mind that we are talking about one tablet. A bottle containing a month's supply would require 30 times that amount. Finally, that is just one vitamin. You'd have to pull off equally implausible feats to supply all the other nutrients in your multivitamin or B complex supplement. The bottom line is that "all natural" supplements where all the vitamins and minerals come from whole foods are a physical impossibility. If the company lies to you about that, they are probably lying to you about other things as well.

Of course, there are some companies that will be only too happy to agree that folic acid is synthetic. They sell methylfolate supplements, and their claim is that methylfolate is natural, while folic acid is not. They claim their methylfolate came from whole foods, not a chemical plant. That is an equally preposterous claim. It would take just as many cups of lentils, spinach, etc. to provide an RDA amount of methylfolate as it would to provide 400 micrograms of folic acid.

So where does all that methylfolate come from? Most of it is manufactured by Merck and Pamlab, the **nutraceutical** division of Nestle. When you look at their patent[2] you discover that it is a purely chemical synthesis starting with folic acid, so there is absolutely no way that methylfolate could be more natural than folic acid. Once again deceptive marketing has trumped integrity.

Natural vs Synthetic

If the "all natural" claim is bogus, are there really any differences between natural and synthetic supplements? I would argue that the answer to that question is Yes. There are, in fact, some very important differences between natural and synthetic supplements. However, because there is no standardized definition of what the term "natural" means, let me define some of the important differences that you should look for in natural food supplements.

#1: Natural food supplements should not contain artificial ingredients. By that I mean they should contain no artificial sugars, colors, flavors or preservatives.

#2: Natural food supplements should supply a full spectrum of nutrients in nature's balance. For example, foods don't just contain pure α-*tocopherol*. They also contain β-, γ-, and δ-tocopherols along with a full spectrum of tocotrienols. Supplements containing pure α-tocopherol may be "natural," but they are incomplete – and that can be a problem. For example. when you take a lot of α-tocopherol, you prevent the absorption of γ- and δ-tocopherol from the foods that you eat.

That is a concern because animal studies suggest that it's the γ- and δ-tocopherols that reduce cancer risk[3]. So consuming large amounts of high purity α-tocopherol might actually increase your risk of cancer. I'm not saying that it does. The jury is still out on that one. But that possibility exists because you're not getting all the naturally occurring tocopherols in balance.

The same is true with B vitamins. One recent study[4] suggested that individual B vitamins may increase your risk of dying, but when you supplement with multiple B vitamins in combination the risk disappears. Similarly, if you are a smoker, beta carotene by itself, without the other naturally occurring *carotenoids*, may increase your risk of cancer[5].

What you really want to do is look for holistic supplements that provide all the naturally-occurring forms of vitamin E in balance, all the naturally-occurring carotenoids in balance, all the major food antioxidants in balance, all the omega-3 fatty acids in balance, and all the B vitamins in balance. Vitamin supplements should not be thought of as a replacement for whole foods, but they should mimic the balance found in whole foods as much as possible.

#3: Finally, although this does not make most people's list of "natural" characteristics, I feel the manufacturers who claim to be natural should be concerned about sustainability. This is perhaps most relevant when you are considering omega-3 sources or other ingredients that come from rare or endangered resources. In addition, if the ingredients come from third world countries, the companies should do their best to assure that Fair Trade practices are in place to protect the farmers from exploitation. Finally, "natural" companies should do everything they can to minimize their carbon footprint.

I have set some pretty high standards for natural supplement, but there are companies that measure up to these standards. I will address what you should look for in terms of quality controls and scientific backing later in this section of the book.

Magical Fruits

Yet another example of slick marketing trumping good science are what I call the "magic fruit" supplements. First it was the acai berry – then mangosteen – then goji. And now it seems like there is a new exotic fruit marketed each month.

And the hype about these exotic fruits is truly amazing. If you listen to the supplement manufacturers you are led to believe that each one of them has unique polyphenols that provide outstanding antioxidant properties and wondrous health benefits. And, of course, there are marvelous testimonials for each one of them (The placebo effect can be as high as 50% for intangibles like energy and well-being).

So, what do the experts tell us? They say that common berries – things like red raspberries, black raspberries, blackberries, blueberries and strawberries – are just as beneficial as the exotic fruits, if not more so. If you would like more information on the health benefits of berries I would highly recommend reading the articles in the February 13, 2008 issue of the Journal of Agricultural Food Chemistry[6] that came from an International Berry Health Benefits Symposium.

The lead article by Navindra Seeram (p627-629) summarized the key findings of the symposium. Dr. Seeram described the polyphenol composition and antioxidant potential of berries. He also summarized the evidence that berry consumption decreases the risk of many diseases – and slows the aging process.

So, what is the bottom line for you? We know that diets high in fresh fruits and vegetables substantially decrease the risk of diseases like heart disease, diabetes, and cancer. And we also know that of the many fruits that are part of a healthy diet, berries are superstars. They are chock full of vitamins, minerals and polyphenols. They are also antioxidant powerhouses.

And the evidence supporting the health benefits of berries is at least as strong as, if not stronger than, the evidence for the health benefits of those exotic fruits that you've been hearing about.

That is precisely why the experts are telling us that we don't need to go to South America or the South Pacific to find the perfect fruits. We don't need to purchase expensive supplements to get the polyphenols in those "magic fruits." Magic fruits are growing in our own backyards! They are available in your local farmer's market or supermarket.

Water Is Water

It's bad enough that some people are paying a premium price for bottled water that isn't required to be any better than tap water, but the latest fads appear to be things like "alkaline" water and "ionized" water. And these "super" waters come with a hefty price tag.

If you believed the hype behind these products, you would think they are revolutionary advances that will cure all sorts of ills. But the truth is that these enticing claims are completely bogus. They contradict the basic laws of chemistry and biochemistry. More importantly, there are no good quality clinical studies showing that they work!

What Is Alkaline Water?

Let's start with alkaline water – but first a bit of background information. Pure water has a pH of around 7, which is neutral. However, if the water is exposed to air for any length of time it picks up CO_2 from the atmosphere. The CO_2 dissolves in the water and is converted to carbonic acid making most sources of pure water slightly acidic. On the other hand, if metal salts are dissolved in the water it generally becomes slightly alkaline.

The questions we might ask are:

1) Does alkalinizing the body have any health benefits?

In the 1930s Otto Warburg, one of the founders of modern biochemistry, showed that cancer cells were much more dependent on glucose (blood sugar) as an energy source than were most other cells in the body and that cancer cells metabolized glucose in a way that made the cancer cells very acidic.

That information languished for many years, but interest in the "Warburg Hypothesis" has been revived in recent years by cell culture studies showing that cancer cells can be selectively killed by limiting their source of glucose.

In theory, making the body more alkaline would also slow the growth of the cancer cells. There is some evidence to support that hypothesis, but the evidence is still relatively weak. It is the same with the other proposed health benefits of alkalinizing the body. There is some evidence in the literature, but it is not yet convincing. As a scientist I'm keeping an open mind, but I'm not ready to "bet the farm" on it.

2. Can alkaline water alkalinize the body?

Here the answer is a clear-cut NO! In fact, this hypothesis wins one of my "Flying Pig" awards! The body has a very strong buffer system and some elaborate metabolic controls to maintain a near-constant neutral pH. More importantly, water is such a weak buffer that it has almost no effect on body pH!

If you really want to alkalinize your body you can do that by eating more of the alkaline foods (most fruits, including citrus fruits, and most vegetables (except the starchy vegetables), peas, beans, lentils, seeds and nuts) and less of the acidic foods (grains, especially refined grains, meat, especially red meat, fish, poultry and eggs).

I've seen some experts recommend 60% alkaline foods and 40% acidic foods. I can't vouch for the validity of that recommendation in terms of the benefits of alkalinizing the body, but there are lots of other good reasons to eat more fresh fruits and vegetables and less red meat and refined carbohydrates.

Is Ionized Water Beneficial?

Ionized water is an even sillier concept from a chemical point of view. It is very difficult to ionize pure water and the ions that you do create quickly recombine to give you pure water again without any change in pH or physical properties.

If you add sodium chloride (table salt) to the water, you can get electrolysis that creates a slightly alkaline pH at one electrode and a slightly acidic pH at the other electrode. However, as soon as you turn off the current, these pH changes rapidly disappear. Even if you were somehow able to capture some of the alkaline or acidic water, remember that water alone has almost no effect on body pH.

Never Underestimate The Placebo Effect

But what about all those glowing testimonials that you have heard? Once again, you need to remember that the placebo effect is near 50% when it comes to pain relief or a feeling of well-being. You can't repeal the laws of chemistry and bio-chemistry. Water is, after all, just water! Good science trumps good testimonials any day.

The Bottom Line

1) Don't waste your money on alkaline water or ionized water. Water is a very poor buffer and has almost no effect on the pH of our bodies.

2) There may be some health benefits to keeping our bodies in a more alkaline state, but the best way to do that is to eat more alkaline foods and less acid foods (for more information, go to http://www.webmd.com/diet/alkaline-diets).

7 Easy Ways To Spot Fad Diets

Perhaps the best way to end a chapter on the "Lies Of The Food Industry" is to talk about fad weight loss diets. I think it was P. T. Barnum who said: "There is a Sucker Born Every Minute." That's particularly true in the diet world where hucksters seem to be all around us.

You've seen the weight loss ads touting:

- Pills or powders that suppress your appetite or magically prevent you from absorbing calories.

- Fat burners that melt the pounds away.

- New discoveries (juices, beans, foods) that make weight loss effortless.

- The one simple thing you can do that will finally banish those extra pounds forever.

You already know that most of those ads can't be true. You don't want to be a sucker. But, the ads are so compelling:

- Many of them quote "scientific studies" to "prove" that their product or program works.

- Their testimonials feature people just like you who are getting fantastic results from their program. [You can do wonders with "computer enhanced" photographs.]

- Many of those products are endorsed by well-known doctors on their TV shows or blogs. [It is amazing what money can buy.]

So, it is easy to ask yourself: "Could it be true?" "Could this work for me?" Fortunately, the Federal Trade Commission (FTC) has stepped up to the plate to give you some guidance. They have issued a list of seven claims that are in fact too good to be true. If you hear any of these claims, you should immediately recognize it as a fad diet and run the other direction.

Here are the seven statements in ads that the FTC considers as "red flags" for fad diets that should be avoided.

1) Causes weight loss of two pounds or more a week for a month or more without changing your diet and exercise routine.

2) Causes substantial weight loss no matter what or how much you eat.

3) Causes permanent weight loss without lifestyle change even after you stop using the product.

4) Blocks absorption of fat or calories to enable you to lose substantial weight.

5) Safely enables you to lose more than 3 pounds per week for more than 4 weeks.

6) Causes substantial weight loss for all users.

7) Causes substantial weight loss by wearing a product on your body or rubbing it on your skin.

I'm sure you have heard some of these claims before. You may have been tempted to try the products or program. You should know that the FTC said that it considers these to be "Gut Check" claims that simply can't be true.

The Bottom Line: There are no magical pills or potions that will make the pounds melt away. You need to change your diet, change your activity level and make significant lifestyle changes if you want to achieve long-term weight control.

Summary

In this chapter I've given you a few examples of the myths, lies and deceptions that abound in the food and food supplement industries. I've just scratched the surface. New deceptive claims and bogus products appear on an almost daily basis. It is truly buyer beware.

You need to rely on common sense and remember "If it sounds too good to be true, it probably is [too good to be true]." Finally, select food supplement manufacturers with integrity, ones that apply rigorous quality control standards, and ones that have published clinical studies showing their products are both safe and effective.

2

Methylated B's: Myths Or Lies?

How are the lies of the food supplement industry created? Some of them start innocently enough. They are often based on a kernel of truth which is misinterpreted by some well-meaning medical doctors. It's not their fault. We teach future doctors what I call "metabolism light" in medical school. There simply isn't room in the medical curriculum to teach all the details and nuances of human metabolism. We also try to teach them the basics of how to interpret the scientific literature. However, it takes years of experience to get really good at picking out the strengths and weaknesses of clinical studies.

The doctors form their hypothesis and test it on a few patients. If it works, they publish a paper. At that point their idea is picked up by the "sensationalist" bloggers. These are the bloggers who like to focus on the sensational. They delight in writing about "new findings" that go against what the medical profession has been telling you for years. The bloggers don't stop there. They usually expand the claims. They "cherry pick" the scientific literature by quoting only studies that support their viewpoint, and ignoring studies that refute it. In short, they put together a very compelling story. Soon the story is picked up by other bloggers who embellish it further. After it appears on enough sites, people start believing it. A myth is born.

Then supplement companies get in on the act. They sense there is money to be made. They manufacture supplements to provide nutrients supported by the myths. They embellish the mythology even more and put together a compelling story to market their products. This is where the mythology becomes deception. Companies have the responsibility to design their products based on the best science. They have an obligation to tell the truth about their products. They know, or should know, that all their claims are not true. When they make claims, they know cannot be true, they are lying to you.

The saga of methylated B's is a perfect example of how observations based on a kernel of truth became myths and eventually became downright lies. Let me share that story with you.

The Start Of The Methylfolate Story

Let's start with a "kernel of truth" that launched the whole methylfolate saga. It started with a doctor who was having a very difficult time finding a solution for a patient with some significant health issues. The doctor ordered a genetic test and discovered the patient had a deficiency in the $N^{5,10}$-methylenetetrahydrofolate reductase (*MTHFR*) gene. The doctor remembered the reaction catalyzed by MTHFR (shown below), and a light bulb went off. "Eureka," he said. His patient must

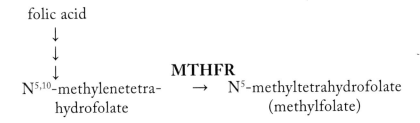

folic acid

$$N^{5,10}\text{-methylenetetra-} \quad \xrightarrow{\text{MTHFR}} \quad N^5\text{-methyltetrahydrofolate}$$
hydrofolate (methylfolate)

be unable to make N^5-methyltetrahydrofolate (commonly referred to as methylfolate), and methylfolate is required for some very important methylation reactions in the cell.

He gave his patient methylfolate, and the patient's symptoms got better. The doctor leapt to the conclusion that other patients with MTHFR deficiency needed methylfolate as well. Many of those patients responded to methylfolate as well. He didn't bother to check whether they would have responded equally well to folic acid. He just assumed methylfolate was the magic elixir. He wrote a paper on his clinical observations, and the methylfolate story was launched.

It all seemed so logical. However, the story was not nearly as straightforward as the doctor and the people publicizing his findings assumed. Let me walk you through some "Metabolism 101." Don't worry. There won't be a quiz.

MTHFR Mutants Only Have a Partial Loss of Activity.

- Individuals with 2 copies of a mutation from A to C at position 1298 of the MTHFR gene (*A1298C homozygotes*) comprise about 5% of the US population. They have 60% MTHFR enzyme activity and appear to be normal in clinical studies.

- Individuals with 2 copies of a mutation from C to T at position 677 of the MTHFR gene (*C677T homozygotes*) have 30% enzyme activity. They comprise about 10% of the US population. C677T homozygotes often have elevated homocysteine levels. The homozygous

C677T mutation is associated with depression, anxiety, and mood swings in some people, but not in others (I will come back to the significance of that qualifying statement later).

- C677T *heterozygotes* (one mutant gene) have 65% activity and are normal.

We Don't Need 100% MTHFR Activity

Our human body is wonderfully designed. For many of our most essential metabolic reactions we have built in redundancy. We don't require 100% activity of key enzymes. This helps protect us from bad effects of mutations as they arise.

The best analogy I can think of is the US space program. Most space vehicles had built-in redundancy so that if one system failed, the mission could go on. For example, you may remember the Hubble space telescope. It was launched with four gyroscopes to keep the telescope pointed in the right direction. After a few years, one gyroscope gave out. That was not a problem because there were three left. A few years later the second gyroscope gave out. Again, there was no problem because there were still two gyroscopes left. It was only after the third gyroscope gave out that Hubble became a bit "wonky," and a space shuttle was sent up to replace the gyroscopes. It is the same with MTHFR. Only when you get down to around 30% activity does the cell become a bit "wonky." (That's about as non-technical as I get.)

Not Everyone With MTHFR Deficiency Experiences Symptoms

This is due to a phenomenon my geneticist friends refer to as *penetrance*. Simply put, that means that not everyone with the same mutation experiences the same severity of symptoms. That is because the severity of a mutation is influenced by diet, lifestyle, and genetic background. Let me start with genetic background. In terms of MTHFR mutants you can think of genetic background as being mutations in a related methylation pathway. People who have a mutation in both MTHFR and a gene in a related pathway will experience more severe symptoms and are more likely to require methylfolate. Once you understand penetrance, you realize why individuals requiring methylfolate represent only a small subset of people who are C677T homozygous.

Penetrance is a concept that most proponents of the methylfolate hypothesis completely ignore. The most severe MTHFR mutation (C677T homozygote) increases the probability that individuals will exhibit symptoms, but some individuals with that mutation are completely normal. Now that you understand the concepts of redundancy and penetrance, you can understand why that is.

When Did The Kernel Of Truth Become A Myth?

Up to this point the hype around methylfolate could be chalked up to an honest misunderstanding. The doctors who published the initial studies may not have known that MTHFR mutations only resulted in a partial reduction in enzyme activity. They probably didn't know the concepts of redundancy (our cells don't need 100% enzyme activity) or penetrance (the same mutation may cause severe symptoms in some patients and have no effect in others). To them it seemed logical to assume that everyone with a MTHFR mutation might do better with methylfolate supplementation. That was incorrect, but it was an honest mistake.

However, the message was picked up by the bloggers who specialize in sensational stories, especially stories that contradict what experts have been telling you for years. They picked up the methylfolate story and distorted it beyond recognition. They knew that "natural" is a buzzword, so they told you that methylfolate was natural and folic acid is synthetic (I exposed that lie in the previous chapter). They told you that methylfolate was better utilized than folic acid. They told you that methylfolate was more effective than folic acid. They told you folic acid was toxic. It was going to increase your risk of heart disease and cancer. Suddenly, the story was no longer about people with MTHFR deficiency. You were being told that everyone should avoid folic acid and use methylfolate instead.

On the surface, these pronouncements should not have passed the "If it sounds too good to be true…" test, or in this case, the "If it sounds too bad to be true…" test. You were being asked to believe that folic acid, which has been in use for over 80 years and is backed by hundreds of studies showing it is safe and effective, was neither safe nor effective. You were being asked to believe that the government was poisoning you by fortifying foods with folic acid.

However, to make their blogs sound more convincing, the bloggers listed clinical studies supporting their stories. The problem is they "cherry picked" the studies that supported their story and ignored the rest. Their bias was particularly outrageous when it came to the "story" that folic acid increases cancer risks. They ignored 10 or 20 studies showing no cancer risk and reported one suggesting it might increase risk. I call that deceptive.

Unfortunately, the myths created by the bloggers have been repeated often enough that many people now believe they are true. I will debunk their myths in a minute, but first let me touch on how their deceptions became downright lies.

When Did The Myths Become Lies?

If you are writing a blog, you are covered by "freedom of speech." You can say whatever you want. It doesn't have to be true. However, if you are a supplement manufacturer, you are held to a higher standard. Ignorance is no longer an excuse. You can no longer cherry pick the "facts" you like and ignore the rest. You are ethically obligated to research all the available literature and be guided by the best scientific evidence.

Reputable companies have been guided by the scientific evidence and have not jumped on the methylfolate bandwagon. They know folic acid is both safe and effective in a wide variety of clinical situations. They also know that, while methylfolate may be just as effective as folic acid, its potential is largely unproven at this point. It has not been tested in many clinical situations. For example, there are dozens of studies showing that folic acid supplementation prior to conception and during pregnancy reduces birth defects. There are zero studies showing that methylfolate reduces birth defects.

Less reputable companies, however, sensed money to be made by capitalizing on the buzz around methylfolate. They repeated the myths of the bloggers to claim that their products were superior to others on the market. They call it marketing. I call it lying. They have an obligation to fact check their claims, and only make claims that are true.

It gets worse. Since lots of people already believed they needed methylfolate, why not extend the claim to methyl B12? That would boost sales even more. The claims for methyl B12 were even more outrageous than for methylfolate. There wasn't even a "kernel of truth" like MTHFR deficiency to serve as a foundation. The claim was that methyl B12 was needed because of some sort of ambiguous "methylation deficiency." The lies had become whoppers.

Debunking The Methylfolate Myths

Now that I have shared the saga of how the methylfolate story progressed from a kernel of truth to myths and eventually to outright lies, let me systematically debunk the myths.

Myth: Methylfolate is natural. It comes from whole food. Folic acid is synthetic.

Fact: I covered this earlier. Methylfolate is chemically synthesized from folic acid. It is physically impossible to extract enough from whole foods to provide 100% of the DV.

Myth: Methylfolate is better utilized by the body than folic acid.

Fact: This claim is based on levels of methylfolate in the blood after taking supplements providing equivalent amounts of methylfolate and folic acid. However, methylfolate has no biological activity in our blood. The measurement that matters is total folate levels (methylfolate plus other folates) in our cells. If you take equivalent amounts of folic acid and methylfolate, you end up with identical folate levels in your cells[7]. In short, there is no difference in our ability to utilize methylfolate and folic acid.

Myth: If you have a mutation in the MTHFR gene, folic acid isn't effective.

Fact: MTHFR slightly increases the need for folic acid (from 400 mcg to between 600 to 800 mcg), but multiple studies show that folic acid supplementation is effective in people with MTHFR mutations. For example, homocysteine levels are easily measured and are a reliable indicator of methylfolate status. One study has shown that folic acid and methylfolate were equally effective at lowering plasma homocysteine in people who were MTHFR C677T homozygotes[8]. That study also showed that folic acid was more effective than methylfolate at lowering homocysteine in people who were C677T heterozygotes and in people with normal MTHFR activity. Another study showed that folic acid was just as effective as a diet providing equivalent quantities of folate from foods at lowering homocysteine levels in people with various MTHFR mutations[9].

At present, lowering of homocysteine levels is the only indicator of methylfolate status for which methylfolate and folic acid have been directly compared. However, there are other studies suggesting that folic acid is likely to be effective for people with MTHFR defects.

For example, folic acid has been shown in multiple studies to be effective in preventing neural tube defects[10], which are highly associated with the C677T MTHFR gene defect. Three studies have shown that supplementation with folic acid, B12, and B6 slowed cognitive decline in older people with elevated homocysteine levels[11-13]. In contrast, the one study that substituted methylfolate for folic acid showed no effect[14].

Myth: Folic acid causes cancer.

Fact: The studies suggesting that folic acid supplementation might increase the risk of cancer were all "outliers." By that I mean they contradicted many other studies showing no increased risk. You may recall that one of "the secrets only scientists know" I shared with you in "Slaying the Food Myths" is that studies sometimes come up with conflicting results. In some cases, we can point to an error in experimental design or statistical analysis as the cause of the aberrant results. In other cases, we never know the reason for the differences, so we go with the weight of experimental evidence (what the majority of studies show). The weight of evidence clearly supports the safety of folic acid.

However, that is sometimes not enough. If there is the slightest possibility that something causes cancer, it demands further investigation. Consequently, the scientific community followed up with larger studies. Those studies showed either reduced cancer risk or no difference in cancer risk with folic acid supplementation. None of the studies found any evidence that folic acid increased cancer risk. I will cover this in detail in section 2 of this book. Of course, the bloggers and the companies selling methylfolate supplements ignored the follow-up studies. The myths and the lies continued.

Myth: Folic acid supplementation during pregnancy increases autism risk.

Fact: This myth is based on a recent study presented at an international meeting. There are two important things you should know about this myth.

#1: This study has not yet gone through the peer review process necessary for publication. We do not know if it is a valid study.

#2: The authors of this study are desperately trying to correct the misleading information that is being circulated about their study. They say their study does not apply to women taking a prenatal supplement containing folic acid during pregnancy. In fact, several studies show that supplementation with 400 mcg of folic acid during pregnancy decreases autism risk. The authors emphasize that the increase in autism risk in their study was only seen in women with 4 times the recommended levels of folate in their blood at delivery. In other words, it only applies to women taking mega-doses of folic acid during pregnancy. I do not recommend taking mega-doses of any vitamin during pregnancy. Furthermore, the risk of autism was correlated with folate levels in the blood, not with folic acid intake. That suggests that mega-doses of methylfolate are just as likely to be problematic as mega-doses of folic acid.

Unfortunately, the best efforts of the authors have not deterred irresponsible bloggers and journalists from spreading the myth that folic acid supplementation at recommended levels during pregnancy may cause autism. That is incredibly bad advice, because multiple studies have shown folic acid supplementation during pregnancy reduces the risk of birth defects.

Myth: Folic acid can mask a B12 deficiency.

Fact: True but irrelevant if you use a supplement with folic acid and B12 in balance.

For more details and references, watch my "Truth About Methylfolate" video in the Video Resources section of **https://healthtipsfromtheprofessor.com**.

Debunking The Methyl B12 Myths

Along with the methylfolate myths have come the methyl B12 myths. Some supplement manufacturers are now claiming that methyl B12 (methylcobalamin) is more natural and more effective than the cyanocobalamin that has been used in supplements for the past 70 years. The arguments are essentially the same as for methylfolate, so let me briefly debunk the methyl B12 claims as well.

Myth: Methyl B12 (methylcobalamin) is more natural than cyanocobalamin. We get the methyl B12 in our supplements from foods.

Fact: As with methylfolate, it would be impossible to extract enough methylcobalamin from foods. In fact, most of the methylcobalamin in supplements is chemically synthesized from either cyanocobalamin or hydroxycobalamin. It can never be more natural than its starting ingredients. A small amount of methylcobalamin is made from genetically modified bacteria.

Myth: Cyanocobalamin is toxic because it contains cyanide.

Fact: You get much more cyanide from common foods such as almonds, lima beans, any fruit with a pit such as peaches, and even some fruits with seeds such as apples. For example, a single almond contains 200 times more cyanide than a supplement providing the RDA of cyanocobalamin.

Myth: Because methylcobalamin is one of the active forms of B12 inside cells (adenosylcobalamin is the other), it is better utilized by cells than cyanocobalamin.

Fact: Cyanocobalamin and methylcobalamin are equally well absorbed by the intestine and equally well transported to our cells. At the cell membrane, the cyano and methyl groups are stripped off and cobalamin (B12) binds to a transport protein called transcobalamin II. Once inside the cell either a methyl group or adenosyl group is added back to cobalamin. In short, methylcobalamin offers no advantage over cyanocobalamin because its methyl group is removed before it enters our cells. Once the methyl and cyano groups have been removed, the cell has no way of knowing whether B12 started out in the methyl or cyano form.

Myth: Methylcobalamin is better utilized than cyanocobalamin for people with methylation defects.

Fact: A methylation defect would affect methylation of cobalamin once it is released from transcobalamin II inside the cell. Because the methyl and cyano groups are removed before cobalamin binds to transcobalamin II, methylcobalamin offers no advantage over cyanocobalamin.

Summary: MTHFR mutations only result in partial loss of activity. Most individuals with MTHFR defects remain symptom free with the RDA, or slightly above the RDA, of folic acid. However, there may be some individuals with a MTHFR defect and additional gene defects in metabolic pathways involving methylation who might benefit from methylfolate. This is due to a phenomenon that geneticists call penetrance and would likely represent a small subset of the population with MTHFR defects. The claims that everyone would benefit from methylfolate instead of folic acid are false. They are contradicted by human metabolism and published clinical studies.

The claims that everyone would benefit from methylcobalamin (methyl B12) instead of cyanocobalamin are even more outrageous. Anyone who takes the time to research how B12 enters our cells would realize that the claim is biochemically impossible.

In short, folic acid has been used for over 80 years and cyanocobalamin for 70 years. There are hundreds of clinical studies showing they are safe and effective, even in most individuals with a MTHFR deficiency. We simply do not know whether methylfolate and methyl B12 will be as effective. For example, there are dozens of studies showing that folic acid supplementation and/or food fortification with folic acid dramatically reduce the prevalence of neural tube defects in newborns. There are zero studies looking at the effectiveness of methylfolate at reducing neural tube defects.

I can't tell you whether the companies selling methylfolate and methyl B12 are ignorant of basic metabolism and the published studies refuting their claims or whether they are purposely trying to deceive the public – but neither is a good thing.

How Can You Protect Yourself From The Lies Of The Food Supplement Industry?

In Chapters 1 and 2, I have given you many examples of the lies of the food supplement industry. I have also given you some advice on how not to be duped by those lies. Let me summarize it here:

#1: Use your common sense. This will be a recurring theme throughout this section of the book. In some cases, it just sounds too good to be true. Claims that all the vitamins and minerals in a supplement are extracted from whole foods fall into this category. In other cases, it just sounds too bad to be true. Claims that the forms of folic acid and B12 that have been proven to be safe and effective in hundreds of clinical trials and are recommended by the Food and Nutrition Board of the National Academies of Sciences and the FDA are dangerous fall into the second category.

#2: **Ignore the hype.** Every company has a compelling story about their products. They hire the very best marketers. It is a shame they don't also hire the best scientists.

#3: **Ignore the testimonials.** Most are fake. Some are genuine but are based on the placebo effect.

#4: **Ignore the endorsements.** Endorsements are bought and sold. Many endorsements are by doctors you have never heard from. I have a perspective on that. I taught medical students for 40 years. Most of the students I taught turned out to be intelligent, dedicated, and compassionate doctors. However, one-third of doctors graduated in the lower third of their class...and that worries me more than it worries you. Occasionally, you will find endorsements by well-known doctors. However, you should be skeptical about those endorsements as well.

#5: **Ask for proof, and ignore junk science.** This is the toughest thing to do. Many companies will use "smoke and mirrors" to try to convince you their products are backed by sound science. I will cover this in Chapter 4 and give you guidelines on how to distinguish between junk science and real science.

3

What Quality Controls?

Every company will tell you that their quality controls are second to none. They will claim that their products are pure and unadulterated. They will swear that what's on the label is in the product. Unfortunately, the truth is often far different.

Quality control tests are expensive. They increase the cost of the product, and they decrease profits. Some companies don't bother with quality control at all. Others farm their manufacturing out to independent contractors and simply assume that what the contractors provide them is pure. It is a very rare company indeed that tests their raw ingredients for purity and potency, sets rigid quality control standards for the manufacturing process, and tests the final product to make sure those standards have been met.

However, the most important decision comes when a final product fails one of those tests. By that time the company will have spent thousands of dollars on the ingredients and the manufacturing process. If the product isn't going to kill anyone, it is all too tempting to just send it out into the marketplace and vow to do better next time. It is only the most ethical of companies that are willing to throw out the substandard product and start over.

Just in case you think these are hypothetical concerns, let me give you some concrete examples:

The FDA has published analyses showing that:

- 60% of ginseng products are worthless because they contain no active ingredients.

- Many garlic supplements also contain no active ingredients. (The easiest way to make a garlic product odorless is to remove the active ingredients.)

Consumer Labs has reported that:

- 90% of chondroitin supplements were worthless because the active ingredient either wasn't present or couldn't be absorbed by the body.

- 37% of saw palmetto products were unacceptable either because the active ingredient was missing or because the product was contaminated.

- 50% of ginseng was contaminated with lead or pesticides.

- USP, GMP, and Standardized Extract on the label meant nothing.

The last statement by Consumer Labs was the most troubling of all, because these are label claims that you should be able to trust. For example:

- **USP** is supposed to mean that a product is pure, potent and easily absorbed by the body. Consumer Labs found products with USP on the label that couldn't be absorbed by the body.

- **GMP** is supposed to mean that a product has been manufactured with the type of quality control tests I described earlier. Consumer Labs found products with GMP on the label that were either contaminated or had no active ingredient.

- **Standardized Extract** applies to herbal products and is supposed to mean that the herbal extract contains the correct amount of active ingredient and that it does not contain contaminants. Again, Consumer Labs found products with Standardized Extract on the label that were either contaminated or had no active ingredient.

Now you know the truth. While everyone claims that their quality control standards are second to none, objective third party analyses show that many of them are lying. That is why any time you hear about a product that contains contaminants or lacks an important ingredient you have to ask: "Did they not know, or did they not care?"

In this chapter, I will give you just a few more examples of the kinds of quality control problems that plague the food supplement industry. At the end of the chapter I will share some questions you should be asking your favorite supplement company about their quality controls.

Who Is Testing Your Supplements?

It's so tempting. You've been getting your supplements from a company that you know and trust – a company that does clinical studies on their products and performs rigorous quality controls. You know their products are pure, safe and effective...

BUT...

You are shopping in your favorite drug store or discount store and you see the same supplements for just a couple of dollars! You can't help thinking, "Wow! Here's the same stuff I've been taking for a lot less money. Why not save my money? They must have run some quality control tests on their products. After all, how bad can they be?"

The answer is:

"Pretty bad!" Here are a few recent examples.

On March 2nd, 2010, the makers and sellers of fish oil supplements were sued by the Mateel Environmental Justice Foundation in California for not telling consumers that their products contained toxic levels of PCBs.

I find it amusing, and somewhat scary, that the FDA did not initiate this action and force the manufacturers to take their contaminated products off the shelves. Instead an environmental consumers group had to sue them for not including PCBs on the label! They sued them under California proposition 65 which requires a warning label whenever a product contains toxic ingredients. In essence, they were sued for not labeling their products "Fish Oil Plus PCBs."

The defendants in this lawsuit were one of the world's largest producer of omega-3 fish oil, and half a dozen major retail chains that had simply slapped their labels on the products without doing any quality control testing of their own. Even scarier is that many of labels on these products said that the omega-3 supplement was treated to reduce or remove PCBs. As a consumer you were led to believe that they were safe!

The bottom line is that the manufacturer probably didn't test for PCBs and neither did the companies selling their omega-3 supplements to the consumer. As I said before, the alternative – that they tested the products, knew that they were contaminated with PCBs, and sold them to the public anyway – is even worse.

Let me share another example you may have heard about. In early 2015 the New York Attorney General claimed that four of the largest retailers in the state were selling bogus herbal supplements. He ordered the retailers to take a number of herbal supplements off their shelves because almost 80% of them didn't contain the ingredients listed on the label or contained non-listed ingredients.

Specifically, the Attorney General claimed that:

- The ginkgo biloba and St. John's wort supplements that they tested from those stores did not test positive for active ingredients.

- Ginseng and Echinacea supplements also failed their tests.

- In some cases, the Attorney General claimed the supplements contained no organic material. They contained sand instead of active ingredients.

The Attorney General claimed that these and other herbal supplements they tested were bogus. Even worse, they were deceptive and could endanger people's health. For example, people generally use St. John's wort to relieve depression. If the supplement is bogus, they are not just wasting money. Their mental health is also being compromised.

While the Attorney General's announcement was alarming, it was also a bit misleading. It was based on an analytic method called "DNA barcoding." In simple terms, DNA barcoding means that DNA is extracted from the sample and the genetic information in that DNA is compared with the genetic information characteristic of the herbal ingredient.

DNA barcoding is an important analytic test that every manufacturer should use to validate the identity of their herbal raw ingredients. However, DNA is often removed in the process of preparing a herbal extract, so DNA barcoding is not always an appropriate assay to use for validating the quality of the finished product. Assays such as the HPLC/MS are more appropriate for the final product. (HPLC/MS is an analytic method that is the gold standard for identifying and quantifying the chemical composition of the final product. However, it is a very expensive procedure, and many manufacturers do not use it.)

In short, the Attorney General had identified a potential problem with the herbal supplement industry, but further tests were required before we could know how significant the problem actually was. Eventually, most of the products on the shelves of the retail outlets in question were independently tested and passed muster. You might be tempted to say it was "much ado about nothing."

However, the press completely missed the scariest part of the story. When the retailers challenged the Attorney General's analysis of their products, the Attorney General replied, "Prove it. Send me your Certificate of Analysis." It turns out that many of the retailers had not done quality controls on their products. When they asked their suppliers for a Certificate of Analysis, the suppliers responded: "You never asked us to run any quality controls. We don't have a Certificate of Analysis." These were major retailers the public was trusting with their health, but they had no idea what was in the supplements they were selling. It truly is a "buyer beware" world.

It gets even scarier. Have you ever wondered what happens when a company does perform quality controls and rejects a raw ingredient or a finished product? In October 2017, the American Botanical Council revealed one of the industry's dirty little secrets when they proposed a plan to require that all rejected ingredients and products be destroyed. That sounds logical. If you were like me, you probably assumed that was already the industry standard.

However, according to the American Botanical Council, the current practice is for companies to return the rejected material to the supplier. In fact, they have to do that if they want to get their money back. The supplier then turns around and sells the material to another company that either doesn't run quality controls or doesn't care. According to the Executive

Director of the American Botanical Council: "That's what's happening. We all know it. Rejected material stays in the supply chain."

What Does This Mean For You?

There are reputable companies who run extensive quality controls and whose products you can trust. Unfortunately, there are also companies who run few, if any, quality controls. You don't know whether their products contain the ingredients on the label, and you don't know if their product is contaminated. Even worse, these companies often use ingredients that reputable companies have rejected. I will help you learn how to recognize the companies you can trust at the end of this chapter. First, let me give you a few more examples of quality control disasters.

Would You Like Some Arsenic With Your Kelp?

In my book, "Slaying The Food Myths," I warned you about arsenic and lead in rice protein because of groundwater contamination. Unfortunately, it's not just rice protein that may be contaminated with heavy metals. Here is another example.

If a waiter in a restaurant asked you: "Would you like some arsenic with your kelp?", you would think that he was crazy. Yet a report[15] published in 2007 suggested that many kelp supplements on the market may be contaminated with arsenic.

The story starts with a 54-year-old California woman using kelp supplements who reported a two-year history of hair loss, fatigue and memory loss. Her primary care doctor couldn't find anything wrong with her and told her that her symptoms were probably related to menopause. Since conventional medicine had not given her a diagnosis or treatment, she increased her intake of kelp supplements hoping that would help.

Over the next several months the woman's short- and long-term memory became so impaired that she could no longer remember her home address. She also reported having a rash, nausea and vomiting, which made it very difficult to work and forced her to leave a full-time job. At that point her doctors became suspicious of arsenic poisoning. Tests revealed high levels of arsenic in her blood and urine. Tests also revealed high levels of arsenic in her kelp supplement. The doctor told her to discontinue the kelp supplement and in a few weeks her symptoms disappeared.

The doctors then purchased 9 different kelp supplements from local health food stores and sent them to a lab to be analyzed. 8 of the 9 were contaminated with arsenic and 7 had arsenic levels that exceeded the tolerance levels for arsenic in food products set by the U.S. Food and Drug Administration (FDA).

What is the bottom line for you? Most of you probably aren't using kelp supplements. In fact, I can't think of any good reason to take kelp supplements. However, this is just another reminder that "nobody's minding the store." Many manufacturers don't perform even the most rudimentary quality control tests, and the FDA is simply overwhelmed. They don't have the resources to test every product on the market. When products like this slip through the safety net, we are the ones who pay with our health.

The Red Yeast Rice Bust

The woman in the previous story probably assumed that her kelp supplement was safe because it was natural. However, just because a supplement is natural doesn't necessarily mean that it is either safe or effective. Red yeast rice is a perfect example. Many people think of red yeast rice as a natural alternative to statins for reducing cholesterol levels. They also believe red yeast rice side effects are non-existent. Nothing could be further from the truth!

The active ingredients in red yeast rice are a class of compounds called monacolins, which are close analogs of the statin drugs. In fact, the most abundant monacolin, monacolin K, is identical to the statin drug lovastatin. That destroys one myth. If a red yeast rice product contains as much monacolin K as a lovastatin pill, it would have the same benefits – and the same side effects.

It only gets worse! In fact, you have no way of knowing how much monacolin K is in your red yeast rice supplement. Because lovastatin is a drug, manufacturers are caught in a Catch-22 situation. If the manufacturers were to actually standardize and disclose the levels of monacolin K in their product, the FDA would consider it an unapproved drug.

When manufacturers don't standardize their active ingredients, bad things happen. How bad, you might ask? A recent study[16] analyzed the concentration of active ingredients in 12 commercially available red yeast rice supplements. The results were appalling:

- Total monacolins in the supplements ranged from 0.31 to 11.15 mg/ capsule.

- Monacolin K (lovastatin) ranged from 0.10 to 10.09 mg/capsule. To put that into perspective, therapeutic doses of lovastatin range from 10 to 80 mg/day.

It gets even worse! The study also measured levels of a toxin called citrinin that is produced by a fungus and is potentially toxic to the kidneys. This is not a toxin that you would find in a pharmaceutical product like lovastatin, but it was present in high levels in one-third of the red yeast rice formulations tested.

To sum it all up, if you were to go out and purchase a red yeast rice supplement:

- You might get a batch with no active ingredients. It wouldn't have any of the side effects of a statin drug, but it wouldn't have any efficacy either.

- You might get a batch that would have the same efficacy and the same side effects as a low dose statin drug.

- You would have a 33% chance of getting a batch that was contaminated with a toxin that you would never find in a statin drug – one that might damage your kidneys.

I don't know about you, but after reading that study I have no desire to ever try a red yeast rice supplement.

Are Herbal Supplements Bogus?

Unfortunately, sometimes mislabeled products aren't simply due to poor quality controls. Sometimes, the adulteration is on purpose. For example, in mid-January 2015 the headlines claimed that most supplements containing grape seed extract were bogus.

The headlines about supplements containing grape seed extract were based on a study[17] by botanical and medicinal chemistry experts at Rutgers University. They obtained 21 commercially available supplements containing grape seed extract from vitamin supplement retailers, supermarkets and online vendors.

The scientists used HPLC/MS to analyze the supplements for the polyphenols that should be found in authentic grape seed extracts. (Again, HPLC/MS is the gold standard for identifying and quantifying the chemical composition of the final product.) The results of their analysis were quite alarming.

- Only 6 of the 21 products tested had the specific polyphenols found in authentic grape seed extract in the amount specified on the label.

- 9 of the products had less than 15% of the polyphenols found in grape seed extract.

- 5 of the products had less than 3% of the polyphenols found in grape seed extract.

- One of the products had no detectable grape seed extract polyphenols.

- 9 of the products contained polyphenols that were characteristic of peanut skin extracts rather than grape seed extract. Peanut skin extract is a much cheaper source of polyphenols than grape seed extract. Substitution of peanut skin extract for grape seed extract is a concern because:

    o While polyphenols from peanut skin extract may have health benefits, they have not been tested. There is currently no clinical evidence that they are beneficial.

    o There is no label information on the products indicating that peanuts were used in their manufacture. This could be a concern for people with peanut allergies.

- 3 of the products contained polyphenols that were more characteristic of pine bark extract than grape seed extract. Again, this is a concern because that blend of polyphenols has not been shown to provide the same health benefits as grape seed extract.

The authors of this study concluded that "adulteration of grape seed extract in commercial preparations is a significant problem." This kind of adulteration is not accidental. You don't start out with peanut skin or pine bark extract and expect to end up with grape seed extract. The authors suggested that substitution of much cheaper polyphenol sources such as peanut skin extract or pine bark extract offered significant "economic gain" to the manufacturers.

They went on to say: "due to reliance of inferior…assays [or complete lack of quality control assays in some cases] across the value chain, adulteration can go undetected by others in the distribution chain, such as those involved in distribution, packaging, wholesale and retail sales."

To put that in lay terms, it means that suppliers and manufacturers often cheat by substituting cheaper polyphenol sources, primarily for financial gain. Furthermore, because most companies don't use high-cost quality control assays such as HPLC/MS, they have no idea whether their products actually contain grape seed extract or not.

You already knew that it is "buyer beware" in the food supplement industry. But after reading about studies like this, you are probably asking yourself "Is it really this bad? Are most herbal supplements a waste of money? How can I be sure that I am getting my money's worth when I buy herbal supplements?" I will give you guidelines at the end of this chapter for selecting manufacturers and products you can trust.

You Can't Always Believe What They Say

At the beginning of this chapter I told you the obvious: Every supplement manufacture will tell you they manufacture their products to the highest quality control standards. You probably already knew that not all of them were telling the truth. How else could you explain the investigative reports that I have shared with you showing that some supplements picked up at random from health food stores or purchased over the internet have serious contamination problems, no active ingredient, or even the wrong ingredient?

If every supplement manufacturer who lied to us about their quality controls grew a long nose like Pinocchio, it would be easy to choose a quality supplement, but in real life things just don't work that way. However, the good news is that the FDA, after years of inaction, is finally starting to inspect the manufacturing facilities of some of these companies and is taking steps to put the really bad players out of business.

Of course, the bad news is that the FDA doesn't have nearly enough inspectors to inspect the many thousands of manufacturing facilities in the United States. In addition, inspecting manufacturing facilities is not the FDA's top priority. Their #1 priority is identifying and shutting down companies that purposely manufacture products that are dangerous. Their #2 priority is shutting down companies that make illegal health claims or claims based on bogus science. (I will discuss both of those topics later in this section of the book.) Inspecting manufacturing facilities to make sure that appropriate quality controls are in place and there is no adulteration of their products is a distant third on their list of priorities.

Even worse, whenever the FDA shuts them down, the really bad players in the industry just reopen under a different name. I call this the "Whack A Mole" effect after the carnival game of the same name. The FDA is doing its best, but it is clearly over-matched. Plus, if you happen to buy a product manufactured in another country, you may be out of luck. Nobody is monitoring the manufacturing facilities for some of the supplements that are made outside of the US.

Quality Claims Versus Reality

Let's go back to the main question – can you really believe the claims of product quality made by every one of the supplement manufacturers? I came across a recent report about an FDA action against a supplement company based in upstate New York that suggests the answer to this question is a clear no.

The company in question states on their website: "Our quality products begin with the purchase of the finest ingredients and packaging materials from carefully selected suppliers.

Incoming raw materials undergo stringent quality control inspections for potency and purity to assure conformance to the product specifications. Careful storage and handling of raw materials maintain optimal viability of all components."

That sounds pretty good. But in fact, the FDA recently filed an injunction to halt the production and distribution of dietary supplements by that company because of multiple violations of current standards for Good Manufacturing Practices (GMP) in the manufacturing, packaging, labeling and holding operations of their dietary supplements.

Specifically the FDA alleged that this company "failed to conduct appropriate tests or examinations to verify the identity of raw ingredients prior to their use and failed to qualify suppliers of raw ingredients through confirmation of their Certificate of Analyses through tests or exams prior to the use of the ingredients that the suppliers provided." Basically, the FDA is saying that the company failed to live up to its claim that they carry out "stringent quality control tests to assure potency and purity" of the raw ingredients they were using.

The FDA also alleged that this company "failed to use effective measures to protect against the inclusion of metals or other foreign materials in their dietary supplements." In other words, the FDA is saying that they may have introduced contamination into their products in the manufacturing process.

And finally the FDA alleged that this company "failed to hold the individual ingredients of the dietary supplements under conditions that do not lead to mix up, contamination or deteriorations of the ingredients as required." In other words, the FDA is saying that the company failed to live up to its claim that they perform "careful storage and handling of raw materials [to] maintain optimal viability of all components."

While these are allegations that ultimately need to be proven in a court of law, it appears likely that the facts may be very different from the quality control claims made by the company. I wish I could tell you that this was an isolated case. But as the FDA is starting to investigate supplement manufacturers, they are finding more and more manufacturers who are cutting corners on product quality to keep their operating costs low. To make matters worse, their marketing claims for quality controls are very different from reality. It is almost impossible for you as a consumer to know whether their quality control claims are true or not.

How Can Consumers Protect Themselves?

Now that you know that some supplements on the market may lack active ingredients or may be contaminated, how do you protect yourself? How do you make sure that you are not wasting your money and jeopardizing your health? The answer is pretty simple:

- Ignore the slick marketing.

- Don't base your decision on price alone.

- Do your research. Ask questions. Only choose reputable companies that do quality controls on both the raw ingredients and the finished product.

The problem, of course, is that every company claims to run stringent quality control tests. My suggestion is to ask them how many quality control tests they run and what kind of tests they run. Here are the questions to ask:

1) Do you run tests to confirm the purity of your raw ingredients, or do you accept the claims of your suppliers? If you do run your own quality control tests on raw ingredients, how many do you run? As described above, some companies do no testing. The industry standard is USP (US Pharmacopeia) screening for about 190 contaminants. The good companies use that. However, the best companies use PAM (Pesticide Analytical

Manual) screening. It is more expensive, but it screens for 350 contaminants.

2) How many quality control tests do you run on your final product? If it is a single nutrient product, the number should be in the dozens. If it is a multivitamin, the number should be in the hundreds. For more complex products, you should expect a thousand or more quality control tests.

3) Do you run quality controls on every batch...or, put another way...How many quality controls do you run each year? Those should run into the tens of thousands.

4) What kind of analytic methods do you use?

- DNA testing (also known as DNA barcoding) is the gold standard for testing the authenticity of the raw ingredients and confirming non-GMO claims. It is a relatively new method in the supplement industry, but should become the industry standard soon.

- HPLC/MS (also referred to as LC/MS) is the gold standard for making sure that the final products contain active ingredients in the proper amount and do not contain contaminants or adulterants. It is expensive, and many companies don't use it.

- ICP/MS is the gold standard for detecting heavy metal contamination. It is even more expensive, and most companies don't use it.

5) Do they test for microbial contamination?

6) What do you do if your product does not meet specifications? You would hope the answer will be "We destroy it."

These are tough questions, but they are the right questions to ask before you pick a supplement company. After all, you are entrusting your health to their products.

4

Junk Science

In this chapter I will focus on the "junk science" many companies use to support their product claims and provide some guidelines to help you distinguish between "junk science" and real science.

I have already alluded to the importance of choosing a company that does clinical studies on their products to assure efficacy and safety. Ideally, those clinical studies should be performed by reputable scientists at major research universities in this country.

"Why is that important?" you might ask. Let me relay my personal experience. My research area was cancer drug development. Because I developed some useful assays for evaluating potential cancer drugs, I was approached by a number of drug companies over the years to test their candidate drugs. Before we could enter into a research contract, the companies were required to sign a contract, drawn up by university lawyers, giving me complete control of the data and publication rights.

I could publish whatever I found, even if it showed the company's drug did not work. They could not edit or block the publication. This is the kind of integrity that is essential if you are going to trust published results.

In years past it was no secret that there were only a few companies that funded and published clinical research studies on their products. Those companies became the "gold standard" of the industry. Of course, it didn't take long for all the other companies to figure out that scientific research was a "point of differentiation" that savvy consumers were looking for, so they decided to copy what the industry leaders were doing. There was just one problem. Clinical research is expensive, and they just didn't want to spend that kind of money.

What do those companies do? They give you "junk science" instead of real scientific studies. By "junk science" I mean studies that sound impressive, but don't really prove anything. I will give you several examples in this chapter, but let me start with an overview:

Many companies will proudly list studies done in test tubes, cell culture, and/or animals and try to convince you those studies prove their products work. I covered that topic in my book, "Slaying The Food Myths," but let me recap briefly here. Studies that are done in test tubes, cell culture, and animals can suggest possible mechanisms of action and give you an idea of what their product might do, but those studies can't really tell you what those products will do for you in your body. If the test tube, tissue culture and animal studies are not backed up by clinical studies in humans, they haven't told you anything of value. You still don't know whether products work in the human body.

Even when the companies do cite clinical studies to back their products, you need to make sure that the studies have been published in peer-reviewed scientific journals because this in another area where unscrupulous companies will cut corners. But before we talk about how companies cut corners, let me try to give you some insight into why the peer review process is so important. As someone who has published over 100 papers in peer-reviewed journals, I am well qualified to describe the process to you.

The peer review process starts when you send your manuscript to a journal. It is first reviewed by an editor. If the editor feels the study might be suitable for their journal, he or she sends it to your competitors (peers) for review.

- If they think your hypothesis is illogical, they will reject it.

- If they think your experimental design is inadequate to test your hypothesis, they will reject it.

- If they think you didn't collect enough data, they will reject it.

- If they think your analysis of the data is improper, they will reject it.

- If they think your conclusions weren't supported by your data, they will reject it.

This is a process that can take weeks or months. When you hear back from the initial review, your manuscript may be rejected. Alternatively, the reviewers may ask you to rewrite sections of your paper, redo your analysis, or even collect more data before resubmitting the manuscript for another review. The closest non-scientific analogy I can think of would be "running the gauntlet." It is a very demanding process, but that is exactly why it is so valuable.

Now that you understand what peer review is, let me give a couple of quick examples of how companies will try to deceive you into thinking they have peer-reviewed studies to back their products.

Many companies will show you what the industry calls "white papers" that they claim prove all the miraculous benefits you can expect from their products. "White papers" are clinical studies done by their scientists or scientists that they hire that have not been published in scientific journals. The charts and graphs may look impressive, but they have never been subject to the rigors of peer review by outside experts. You simply do not know whether you can believe the results.

Another way that some companies evade the peer-review process is to publish in what I call "advertising journals." These are journals with no peer review process. The company pays an "advertising fee" to have their study published. This is the hardest type of sham for the layperson to detect. The study is published in a journal. It looks legit. But, in fact, it is just an advertisement.

In this chapter I will give you specific examples of "white paper" studies, studies published in "advertising journals," and other kinds of junk science you need to look out for when you are evaluating the health claims for any supplement you may be considering.

Junk Science Versus Real Science

It's hard to know who to trust in the food supplement industry. In terms of scientific proof that their products work, I've given you a quick summary of some of the worst abuses in the introduction to this chapter. I'd like to go into a bit more detail here. For example, everyone claims that their product is backed by solid science. But most companies rely on "borrowed science" to back their product.

What do I mean by "borrowed science?" Simply put, they are citing references that show that an ingredient in their product has a desired effect. They aren't actually doing studies with their product. That is critically important because the ingredients in a product interact with each other. They can affect the uptake and utilization of each other in the body. In short, unless you test the final product for safety and efficacy, you really don't know whether it works or not.

Even when the company has clinical studies on their product, you need to look at where those "studies" are published (or not published). Let's start with the studies that aren't published. We call these "white papers." Some companies will tell you that "Our scientists have shown..." My questions are:

- If their scientists hadn't "shown" that the product worked, would they still have a job tomorrow? I never trust studies that are not run by an independent scientist at a major university or research organization.

- If the study was well designed, how come it was never published? If the study was valid, it should be able to stand up to the rigors of peer review that are required for publication in scientific journals.

But just because a company tells you that their study has been published doesn't mean that it's a valid study. As I said in the introduction, there are "advertising journals" that will publish any study that you submit if you pay them enough.

After I first mentioned that fact in a blog post several years ago, I received an email that I thought would be worth sharing with you (the names have been changed to protect the not-so-innocent). The email read:

"You mentioned that many supplement companies will say they have published research in medical journals when in fact the information is published in an advertising journal with a medical-sounding name. I know for a fact that this is true. Let me tell you of a personal experience in 1998. Because of my pharmaceutical and vitamin manufacturing industry background, I have always had to be somewhat of a "sleuth" to uncover which manufacturers are truthful. Because of many industry secrets I uncovered during that previous career, I guess I have become a skeptic.

"In April 1998 an acquaintance of mine here in town participated in a Wellness Expo I organized for my chamber of commerce. She represented XXX Encapsulated Powders that claim to be concentrated fruits and vegetables. She claimed her products had been clinically tested and gave me a copy of a reprint to read entitled "American Medical Review, April 1996, Volume 2, Issue #4." It listed 4 articles on the front cover, but when you opened it there was only a one-page article about XXX. No author, no footnotes, no reference information. Poorly written! It claimed studies had been done by "an independent laboratory" and "a prominent pathologist" but didn't give names, etc. When I told her this was weak information, she said, "Well, look at the name! It's a medical journal! It must be accurate information!"

"So, I called the phone number for this American Medical Review. The receptionist answered the phone "MAY Enterprises." MAY turned out to be the initials of the publisher Mark A.Y. Through my sleuthing, I actually got to talk to Mark (he thought I was a potential advertiser) and he told me the American Medical Review was an advertising journal. NOT A MEDICAL JOURNAL. He told me that if I were looking to publish an article about my company and would agree to his prices and terms, I could publish my proposed article (of course I had made this whole thing up to get him to talk to me)."

Her email says it all! The sad thing is so many companies intentionally mislead their customers, just to make a buck. By the way, you don't have go to the lengths that she did to distinguish between a real scientific journal and an advertising journal. The National Library of Medicine keeps an online database of all scientific journals in the area of medical research (where clinical studies would be published) called PubMed. Just Google PubMed. You'll find it. If the journal isn't listed in PubMed, it's probably an advertising journal.

Shake, Shake...Busted

Perhaps the best way to illustrate what I have just covered is to give you some specific examples. This example is from a few years ago, but you may remember the TV ads. You just shook these "magic" crystals on your food and the pounds would melt away. And, by the way, it was not salads they were shaking the crystals on. It was pizza, hamburgers, French fries and the like.

The "magic" crystals were made from maltodextrin (a carbohydrate derived from starch), tricalcium phosphate, natural and artificial flavors, soy and milk ingredients. The manufacturer claimed that those crystals suppressed appetite and led to weight loss. Supposedly, these claims were supported by two clinical studies showing, for example, that people using the "magic" crystals lost an average of 30 pounds over six months while the control group only lost two.

Now if you think these claims sounded too good to be true, you weren't alone. California District attorneys filed a false advertising lawsuit against the manufacturer of the crystals, and eventually the manufacturer agreed to settle and pay $800,000 in civil penalties and $105,000 in restitution to California consumers.

It turns out that neither of the clinical studies was good enough to be published in a peer-reviewed scientific journal. In addition, the lead researcher for one of the studies admitted in a deposition that she had no scientific training and was not qualified to conduct a nutrition intervention study.

So, a great-sounding ad bit the dust. Of course, there is no magic formula or magic ingredient that will just make the pounds melt away. The physiological equation has not changed. Weight loss occurs when calories out exceed calories in. And permanent weight loss requires lifestyle changes.

Is Green Coffee Bean Extract Bogus?

This example dates back to 2012. The ads were everywhere. They were on the internet, in print, and on TV. Once again, the claims sounded so appealing. You could just take this green coffee bean extract and the pounds would melt away. You didn't need to exercise or change your diet. Your first reaction when you heard those claims was probably "Right, when pigs fly. I've heard this kind of stuff before. It's just too good to be true."

But then you were given a pseudo-scientific explanation about how it was the chlorogenic acid in the green coffee bean extract that was responsible for its amazing properties. (What they didn't tell you was that chlorogenic acid is present in all roasted coffees.) You were told that it was backed by a clinical study showing that people lost 17.7 pounds, 10.5% of their body weight and 16% of their body fat in 22 weeks without diet and exercise.

To top it all off you were told that it was endorsed by Dr. Oz on his TV show and provided with a video clip to prove it. After all of that, you were probably tempted to say "Maybe… just maybe… these amazing claims might be true." You may have even been tempted to try it.

Evidently the Federal Trade Commission did not consider the claims about green coffee bean extract to be true. The FTC sued the company that manufactured and sold green coffee bean extract for promoting a "hopelessly flawed study" to support the weight loss claims for their product.

The FTC alleged that:

- The study was too small, at 16 subjects, to provide convincing data.

- The study contained several critical flaws in its design and results. For example, the greatest weight loss occurred in the placebo group.

- The lead investigator in India falsified the results.

- The company knew or should have known that this botched study didn't prove anything.

The manufacturer eventually agreed to pay $3.5 million to the FTC to settle their complaint. Basically, the company agreed with the FTC that there was no evidence to back their weight loss claims.

How Did Dr. Oz Get It So Wrong?

What about Dr. Oz's endorsement? In Dr. Oz's 2012 show segment he called green coffee bean extract "the magic weight loss cure for any body type." The most puzzling aspect of this whole saga is how Dr. Oz got it so wrong.

After all, he is a trained neurosurgeon. He is Vice Chair of the Department of Surgery at Columbia University. He understands the principles of evidence-based medicine. Evidence-based medicine simply means that it is a physician's responsibility to check the scientific evidence before recommending a treatment to a patient. Yet he never even looked into the supposed "clinical study" backing green coffee bean extract's weight loss claims.

At a Senate hearing in June 2014, Dr. Oz apologized. He said: "For my colleagues at the FTC, I realize I have made their jobs more difficult."

The Fake Chocolate Study

Unfortunately, even publication in a PubMed-listed journal is not always a guarantee that the study is a quality study you can trust. The most egregious example of this is something I call "the fake chocolate study."

The fake chocolate study was a hoax put together by John Bohannon, an investigative journalist and correspondent to

Science (a very well-respected scientific journal), to test the peer review system. The study was real, but it was seriously flawed. For example, it had only 16 subjects, there was no effort made to determine what the subjects were eating other than chocolate, and the conclusions were not supported by the data. In short, it was a very bad study – one that would have been rejected by any reputable journal.

For the purposes of the test he called himself Dr. Johannes Bohannon from the "Institute of Diet and Health," a non-existent entity that consisted of nothing more than a fake website he set up. He then wrote up the study and titled it "Chocolate With High Cocoa Content As A Weight Loss Accelerator" with the conclusion (not supported by the data) that "Long-term weight loss, however, seems to occur easier and more successfully by adding chocolate. The effect of chocolate, the so-called 'weight loss turbo', seems to go hand in hand with personal well-being, which was significantly higher than in the control groups."

In March 2015 he submitted the article to 20 online journals. Several accepted it within 24 hours. He chose to publish it in the "International Archives of Medicine." His paper was published online without any revisions two weeks later. [Note: You should not assume the fact that several of just 20 journals accepted his paper as an indication that a significant percentage of journals accept sub-standard papers without serious peer review. He had, in fact, done previous research for Science magazine identifying those journals most likely to accept flawed studies. It was to those types of journals he sent his fake study.]

John Bohannon was later quoted as saying "Editors of reputable journals reject [these kinds of studies] out of hand without even sending them to peer reviewers. But there are plenty of journals that care more about money than reputation." [It cost him $650 to have his article published in the International Archives of Medicine.]

If this study had just been published in an obscure journal and had been ignored, that would have been bad enough. But the story gets even worse. He then created a press release that he sent to news outlets. The press release made some outrageous statements and even contained a link to an unrelated music video. However, the study made news headlines in more than 20 countries in half a dozen languages. For example, headlines from the Daily Express in England blared: "Chocolate Accelerates Weight Loss: Research Claims It Lowers Cholesterol and Aids Sleep."

John Bohannon's take was: "The key is to exploit journalists' incredible laziness. If you lay out the information just right, you can shape the story that emerges in the media almost like you were writing those stories yourself. In fact, that's literally what you are doing, since many reporters just copied and pasted our text."

For the complete story of how John Bohannon pulled off this hoax, read his blog post[18]. It makes fascinating reading.

How Can You Protect Yourself Against Junk Science?

How can you protect yourself from falling for junk science? How can you avoid wasting your money on products that don't work, or that may even harm your health? I advise starting with a little healthy skepticism.

Be skeptical about the claims. Once again, the old adage: "If it sounds too good to be true, it probably is [too good to be true]" is always good advice.

Be skeptical about the studies. The bottom line is that not all clinical studies are reliable. I realize that it is extremely difficult for a non-scientist to evaluate the validity of clinical studies. My best advice is to go online and see what other experts are saying about the study and the claims. There are several "fact checker" blogs online that focus on careful scientific analysis of product claims and the "studies" that support them. Just be aware that most companies will arrange for phony "positive reviews" to dupe the casual online browser. Companies will also post articles with a title that sounds like it is going to "expose" the product but contain a story line that endorses it. You will need to search out websites with a reputation for fact checking product claims. You should also search for impartial sources (like Web MD, Mayo Clinic, Cleveland Clinic, Harvard Health Letter, NIH, etc.).

Be skeptical about the endorsements. Dr. Oz was not unique. There are far too many examples of well-known doctors who have endorsed bogus product claims on their TV shows or in their blogs. That makes it even more difficult for the layman to separate fact from fiction. Sometimes, they have been paid for the endorsement. Other times, they are simply looking for something novel to feature in their TV show or blog. My advice is to simply ask the question: "Does their blog or TV show feature something novel, something spectacular, and/or something sensational… every single week?"

My belief is that these experts all start out with good intentions. However, to develop a really big audience and keep their audience engaged, they feel pressured to deliver novel and sensational health news every single week. The reality is that there are not advances every single week that are novel, sensational… and scientifically accurate. Eventually, they feel pressured to sacrifice accuracy for novelty.

There are also some very specific questions you should ask that will help you differentiate between junk science and real science. For example:

Has the study been published? I have seen websites and company literature that describe the studies done on their product in glowing detail. They will tell you the study was done by top scientists at a major university. They will show you figures and data that look convincing. They will say this proves their product works. It is all very impressive. However, **if they don't cite a reference for the publication of their paper, don't believe a word of it.** Because the study has not gone through the peer review process, you have no idea whether it is valid or not. It may be complete fiction for all you know.

Is the main author of the study a reputable scientist at a major university? I explained the importance of that earlier. The best way to find this out is to look up the author in PubMed. Their university affiliation and publications will be listed. They should be affiliated with a major university and have dozens or hundreds of publications listed.

Was the study published in a peer-reviewed journal or an advertising journal? I also explained the importance of that earlier. Once again, the best way to find that out is to look up the journal in PubMed. **If the study was not published in a journal listed in PubMed, it was published in an advertising journal. Don't believe a word of it.**

Was the study done in cell culture or animals rather than in humans? This one is a little more difficult. You often can't tell from the title. However, if you Google the citation (journal, year of publication, volume #, and pages), you can find the abstract and that will usually give enough detail for you to figure it out. **If the study was done in cell culture or animals, you have no idea whether it will work in humans.**

Was the study done with their product or were they using "borrowed science?" By "borrowed science" I mean the actual study was done with another company's product or with an ingredient used in their product. In some cases, it is easy to know that they used borrowed science because they will say: "We use ingredient X, which has been shown to" and list the references to support their statement. In many cases, however, you will need to read the methods section to see what was tested in that study. Fortunately, many journals are fully available online nowadays. If they a freely available online, you can check the methods section. **If they used borrowed science, you have no idea whether their product works.**

Do the results of their study support their claims? Perhaps they cite a short-term study showing their product lowers cholesterol and triglycerides and claim their product reduces your risk of heart disease. Or perhaps, they cite a short-term study showing their product lowers blood glucose levels and insulin and claim their product reduces the risk of diabetes. Things like cholesterol, triglycerides, blood sugar, etc., are imperfect indicators of disease risk. If you want to know whether a product reduces disease risk, you need long-term studies looking at health outcomes. Don't misunderstand me. Those are expensive studies. I don't expect companies to fund studies like that with all their products, but good companies should have one or two long-term studies measuring the effect of their products on health outcomes. **In the absence of long-term studies, you have no idea what effect a product will have on your health.**

You are probably looking at this list and saying: "There is no way I will ever do that much research into a product." I realize that. I wanted my list to be comprehensive, but in reality, you will usually only need to go through the top 2 or 3 to identify most of the products backed by junk science.

Finally, if this all seems a little too hard, just let your skepticism guide you. Your "skeptic's alarm" should ring when you hear about magic crystals that will make the calories disappear or a magic ingredient that will melt away the pounds without diet or exercise. I could go on, but I think you get the point.

5

Supplements That Are Dangerous

Up to this point, I have focused on products that promised more than they could deliver. In Chapters 1 and 2, I talked about products that were based on hype and deception. In Chapter 3, I talked about products that were manufactured without proper quality controls. In Chapter 4, I talked about products that were based on junk science. However, in most cases the worst that could happen was that you might waste your money on a worthless product.

However, there are a few supplements on the market that are actually dangerous. Most of these supplements fall into one of four categories – weight loss, sports nutrition, energy, and sexual enhancement. Most companies that produce products in this category are perfectly safe, but there are a few really bad players in this segment of the market. In this chapter I will give you a few examples of truly dangerous products and give you some tips on how to recognize and avoid them.

It's A Jungle Out There

"It's a jungle out there." You've heard that statement before. It is, however, a perfect saying to keep in mind as we discuss companies that make dangerous products. "How dangerous?", you might ask. There are some companies that make products containing dangerous drugs – drugs that can kill you.

How Bad Can It Be?

In case you are wondering, "How bad can it be?", let me share some data with you. A recent report[19] states that between January of 2004 and December of 2012 there were 465 products that were subject to a class I recall by the FDA. A class I recall is for cases in which there is a reasonable probability that use of or exposure to a product will cause serious adverse health consequences or death.

Now here's the scary part: 98% of those recalls were for dietary supplements. The worst offenders were sexual enhancement products (40%), bodybuilding products (31%) and weight loss products (27%). [Note: If you are good at math, you will have noticed that leaves 2% for recalls of all other dietary supplements.] And these weren't all foreign-made products. 74% were manufactured in the United States.

Will Supplements Put You In The Hospital?

That was followed two years later by a study[20] claiming that dietary supplements were responsible for 23,000 emergency room visits and 2,100 hospitalizations every year. That study was based on an extrapolation from 63 hospitals to every hospital in the United States. Some experts consider this to be an overestimation since it is almost 8 times higher than the 3,200 cases/year in the official FDA's Serious Adverse Event Reporting database. However, for the purposes of this article I will accept the 23,000 number.

Here is a breakdown of the hospitalizations:

- 13% of the ER visits were due to allergic reactions. These were seldom serious enough to require hospitalization. This is also a type of problem that is probably unavoidable. Since many food supplements use natural ingredients, some degree of food allergies is to be expected.

- 13% of the ER visits were due to swallowing problems, primarily in people over the age of 65. The preventative measure here is simple. If you or a loved one has difficulty swallowing, choose pills that are small and slick or chewable, or choose powder or liquid supplements.

- 20% of the ER visits were due to adverse effects caused by unsupervised ingestion of the supplements by children. The preventative measure here is also simple. Keep your supplements out of reach of small children – especially if they are chewable or have attractive colors. While the supplements may be perfectly safe when taken as recommended, the unsupervised ingestion of a whole bottle of almost any supplement by a small child is problematic.

- 41% of the ER visits were due to weight loss products (25.5%), energy products (10%), sexual enhancement products (3.4%) and bodybuilding products (2.2%). The most common adverse effect for these products were heart palpitations, chest pain, and irregular heartbeat. As I said before, these are the kinds of supplements you really need to be most careful about.

Putting These Studies Into Perspective

In the case of the first report you should contrast the 465 recalls over an 8-year period with:

- The more than 35,000 deaths/year from properly prescribed medications... and...

- The 8,000 deaths/year in US hospitals due to medication errors[21]

In the case of the second study you can put the 23,000 number of hospitalizations into perspective by considering that:

- It represents about 0.015% of the 150 million people in the US who use supplements.

- It represents about 1% of the emergency room admissions caused by side effects of properly prescribed medications.

In short, these studies over-dramatize the dangers of dietary supplements. Most dietary supplements are quite safe. However, even one emergency room visit due to a dietary supplement is too many – especially if it were to happen to you or a loved one. Consequently, I will analyze specific examples of dangerous supplements in more detail so that I can show you how to recognize and avoid those few supplements that are truly dangerous.

Why Are Dangerous Supplements Even On The Market?

Let's start with the obvious question: Why are weight loss, energy, sexual enhancement and bodybuilding products the ones most likely to be dangerous? To quote Pogo (I'm really dating myself with this quote): "We have met the enemy, and he is us." Here are some examples of what I mean:

- **Weight Loss Products:** We can listen all day long to experts tell us that we need to make lifestyle changes, and we should aim for no more than one or two pounds of weight loss per week. However, for many of us that advice goes in one ear and out the other. We want to lose weight fast, and we want it to be easy.

- **Energy Products:** Many of us are just plain exhausted because our diets are terrible, we are under stress, and we are burning the candle at both ends. We don't want to eat better and change our lifestyle. We want high octane energy, and we want it now.

- **Bodybuilding Products:** The story is similar, especially for males in the 20-34 age range. We want big muscles, and we don't want to wait for the years of workouts it will take to build that kind of physique naturally. We want it now.

- **Sexual Enhancement Products:** ER admissions for sexual enhancement products were 100% male. What does that say about us guys? I won't even go there.

Most supplement manufacturers are ethical and don't make supplements that could harm you. However, there are a few unscrupulous manufacturers who are only too happy to exploit our human weaknesses if they can make a buck in the process. They will give us exactly what we want, even if it kills us.

You have seen the marketing hype for these products. "Pump up your muscles", "Explode your muscles", "Blast your fat", "Annihilate your fat", "Ramp up your energy": The claims leap off the page of the ads for many sports and weight loss supplements.

The easiest way to create products that will burn off weight effortlessly, build muscle rapidly, and give you energy is to add chemically synthesized stimulants in the amphetamine family. In addition to stimulants, some weight loss products use diuretics, and some energy products use dangerous levels of caffeine, both of which can cause problems. Products to increase muscle mass may contain steroids. Sexual enhancement products often use herbal ingredients like yohimbe bark that can be quite dangerous (more about that later in this chapter).

Unfortunately, you can't count on the FDA to protect you. I will give you several examples of that later in this chapter. It's not clear whether the FDA is unwilling to protect us, or if it is overwhelmed. However, it is clear that if we want to avoid dangerous supplements, it is up to us.

What Were They Thinking?

As I said, the less reputable sports supplement manufacturers often add stimulants to their weight loss and bodybuilding products. Stimulants do raise metabolic rate, so they help with weight loss. They have no effect on athletic performance, but the athletes often feel like they have more energy – so they are also popular in bodybuilding products.

All stimulants carry some risk. Even caffeine can be problematic for some individuals, and many sports supplements contain massive amounts of caffeine. But, it is not caffeine-containing sports products that are the most worrisome. It is the sports supplements containing amphetamine-like compounds that are particularly dangerous. These supplements can increase heart rate, increase blood pressure, and cause arrhythmia. They can even kill people.

If you have followed the weight loss and sports supplement industry over the years this should sound very familiar. Ephedra (also called ma huang), an analog of amphetamine, was first developed as a nasal decongestant. However, because it also had thermogenic (increase in metabolic rate) and stimulant effects, it was widely used in weight loss and sports supplements. There was only one problem. It also caused high blood pressure, arrhythmia and death. After it killed a number of people, the FDA finally banned it in 2004.

The DMAA Scandal

Shortly after ephedrine was banned in the United States manufacturers started looking for other amphetamine-like ingredients to add to their weight loss and sports pre-workout supplements. One of the first to come on the market was DMAA. DMAA is short for the chemical dimethylamylamine. It is structurally very similar to amphetamine. Like ephedra, DMAA was originally developed as a nasal decongestant. Like ephedra, it also has thermogenic and stimulant effects, which made it very desirable for weight loss supplements and sports supplements.

Because it is both a stimulant and an amphetamine analog, the World Anti-Doping Agency added DMAA to its prohibited list in 2010 and numerous elite athletes have been disqualified from competition for DMAA use since then. But that did not keep many other athletes from using DMAA supplements.

And that is a concern because, just like ephedra, DMAA is not an innocuous substance. Reported side effects include headache, nausea and stroke. And, like ephedra, it appears that we can add death to the list of side effects associated with DMAA usage. After two US soldiers died following DMAA usage, the US Army and Air Force Exchange Service stores ordered the removal of all products containing DMAA from their shelves. Dr. Michael Kilpatrick, deputy director of Force Health Protection and Readiness Programs with the Office of the Deputy Assistant Secretary of Defense for Force Health Protection and Readiness (don't you love bureaucratic names!) was quoted as saying the products were pulled from the shelves because "We are concerned about reports of heat illness, kidney (and) liver damage, and sudden death in service members who reportedly used products containing DMAA."

What Were They Thinking?

I might have considered this as just another sad example of a sports supplement industry that puts profits ahead of safety and athletes who are willing to take almost any risk to gain an edge. But the story gets much worse.

It turns out that a major retail nutrition chain recalled all products containing DMAA from their stores on US military bases, but continued to sell those same products in all its other stores. And the CEO of the nutrition chain was quoted as bragging that the DMAA military ban had "no impact whatsoever" on their sales. I don't know which was worse – that the nutrition chain continued to sell the DMAA supplements or that people continued to buy them. **What were they thinking?**

The Scandal Worsens

As you might expect, the deaths kept piling up. Several months later the FDA finally acted. It sent a warning letter to all US manufacturers of DMAA-containing products asking them to stop using DMAA as an ingredient in their supplements. All the companies agreed to stop using it except one. That manufacturer claimed that DMAA could be found in geraniums, which is an approved herbal ingredient, so they continued to use it. And the major retail nutrition chain I mentioned above continued to sell their DMAA-containing products in all its non-military stores.

Finally, on April 11, 2013, the FDA issued a strongly worded warning about DMAA. The FDA warning said that by then there had been 86 reports of illnesses and deaths associated with supplements containing DMAA, and the preponderance of scientific evidence showed that DMAA was not a natural constituent of geraniums. The FDA said that they would take all possible means to get DMAA-containing products off the market. A cynic might point out that the

FDA did not act until the night before a high profile exposé on DMAA was scheduled to appear on NBC.

Finally, the manufacturer threw in the towel and said they would reformulate their DMAA-containing products. A cynic might suspect that they would just substitute another stimulant for DMAA, which, in fact, they did.

What about the major retail nutrition chain? They said, "It [DMAA] will be positioned out of stores, probably over the next five or six months as we sell existing inventory." You don't need to be a cynic to interpret that statement. It wasn't until the FDA raided their warehouses and removed all remaining DMAA-containing products that everyone thought that the DMAA story was finally over.

The FDA Falls Asleep Again

Unfortunately, at the time this book was written, the DMAA saga was not over. In fact, the story gets even worse. Since 2013 the FDA has ignored DMAA-containing products. The Human Performance Resource Center, an initiative of the Department of Defense, recently listed 39 products containing DMAA that are still readily available, either online or from retail stores. Even though the FDA has classified DMAA as an illegal ingredient, it is still readily available, and they haven't acted. So, what's the bottom line for you? As I said earlier, it is a jungle out there. Don't fall for the hype and fancy claims. Do your homework, and stick with a company you can trust.

"Whack A Mole I" – Another Dangerous Product Fills The Void

I alluded to the "Whack A Mole" problem the FDA faces in the previous chapter on quality controls. The fact that amphetamines kill people is of little concern to unscrupulous manufacturers. In fact, as soon as one amphetamine-like ingredient is banned, they just reformulate by adding another amphetamine-like ingredient to their product.

For example, a recent paper by a group of scientists in the United States and the Netherlands[22] reported that DMBA (1,3-dimethylbutylamine), another amphetamine-like ingredient that is a close analog of DMAA, was found in at least 12 products marketed to improve athletic performance, increase weight loss and enhance brain function.

DMBA (1,3-dimethylbutylamine) is a synthetic compound that has never been tested for safety in humans, something that the FDA is supposed to require for every new dietary ingredient added to a supplement. Because DMBA is chemically similar to DMAA (1,3-dimethylamylamine), the scientists conducting the study suspected that manufacturers may have started adding it to their products when DMAA was banned.

The scientists surveyed the listed ingredients on all supplements distributed in the United States for any ingredient name that might be a synonym for DMBA. They identified 14 supplements that fit that criterion and analyzed them for the presence of DMBA. 12 tested positive for DMBA.

The authors of the study stressed that DMBA is a synthetic pharmaceutical ingredient, has the potential to cause the same health risks as DMAA, and has never been tested in humans. They stated: "Given the potential risks of untested pharmacologic stimulants, we strongly recommend that manufacturers immediately recall all DMBA in dietary supplements...The FDA and other regulatory bodies should, without delay, warn consumers about the presence of DMBA in [certain] dietary supplements."

The Council for Responsible Nutrition, an industry group, sent a letter to the FDA on September 12th, 2014 urging regulatory action, noting that "it has a similar chemical structure to the banned ingredient [DMAA] and that none of those selling it have filed required "new dietary ingredient" paperwork with the FDA to substantiate its safety." The FDA waited almost a year to respond. Finally, in mid-2015 it sent a warning letter to manufacturers asking them to remove DMBA from their products.

This story is all too familiar. The unscrupulous manufacturers won't remove unsafe ingredients until they are forced to, and the FDA is far too slow to act. Often the FDA doesn't act until the product kills people, as was the case for products containing DMAA.

Label Deception

If you are like me, you are probably outraged that manufacturers would even consider selling products like these. But the story only gets worse. None of the labels listed DMBA as an ingredient. That's probably because DMBA looks enough like DMAA that intelligent consumers might be scared off.

Instead, they listed the ingredient as AMP citrate. They can do that because they are using AMP to stand for 4-amino-2-methylpentane, which is a chemical synonym for 1,3-dimethylbutylamine (DMBA). But that is not the common usage for AMP. To any biochemist, and probably most high school biology students, AMP stands for 5'-adenosylmonophosphate – a normal and harmless cellular metabolite. Citrate is also a normal cellular metabolite.

In short, the manufacturers were purposely masquerading a synthetic and potentially dangerous stimulant under a pseudonym that looks like naturally occurring cellular metabolites. That is shameful!

Lack of Quality Control

But wait, it gets even worse. The scientists analyzed 14 products that had AMP citrate on the label and the amount of DMBA ranged from 0 to 120 mg. Apparently these manufacturers have no quality control process either. That is a huge concern because this ingredient has never been tested for safety in humans. We have no idea how much it takes to harm people!

"Whack A Mole II" – Another Amphetamine-Like Product Hits The Market

Yet another amphetamine-like analog of DMAA called beta-methylphenethylamine (BMPEA) appeared in the sports nutrition marketplace starting around 2011. It is an isomer of amphetamine that was first synthesized in the 1930s. Because it is an analog of amphetamine, BMPEA is classified as a banned substance by the World Anti-Doping Agency. Unfortunately, its story is all too familiar.

The FDA first reported the presence of pharmacological doses of BMPEA in 43% of sports and weight loss supplements containing the herbal ingredient *Acacia rigidula* in 2012. The FDA requested that manufacturers voluntarily remove BMPEA from their products. In response, the manufacturers claimed that the BMPEA in their products was a natural ingredient that came from the *Acacia rigidula*, even though there was no scientific evidence that it had ever been successfully extracted from *Acacia rigidula*.

BMPEA causes high blood pressure in animals and has never been tested for safety or efficacy in humans. However, the FDA did not warn consumers that supplements with the ingredient *Acacia rigidula* might contain BMPEA and might, therefore, be dangerous.

A group led by Dr. Pieter Cohen of Harvard University recently decided to analyze sports and weight loss supplements containing *Acacia rigidula* to see whether companies had voluntarily removed DMPEA from their products over the last two years. One might hope that companies might have been more motivated by protecting the health of their customers than by profit.

Not a chance! Dr. Cohen and his colleagues tested 21 products containing *Acacia rigidula* and found that 11 of them (52%) contained BMPEA – some in amounts as high as 94 mg/serving[23]. Dr. Cohen was quoted as saying "More than two years after the FDA's discovery [of BMPEA in sports supplements], the FDA has yet to warn consumers about the presence of an amphetamine isomer in supplements. This is really about the FDA and why the FDA is not enforcing the law. This is a great example of how the FDA could so easily move now and not wait like it did with DMAA, wait until strokes and heart attacks had become front page news."

After Dr. Cohen's article became front page news, several senators called on the FDA to ban BMPEA. A week later the FDA finally caved in and announced that BMPEA was not a legal ingredient and that any products listing it on the label must be withdrawn from the market. A skeptic might note that this was a full two years after the FDA discovered the existence of products containing BMPEA. Even worse, the FDA's announcement only covered products with BMPEA on the label. It did not cover BMPEA-containing products listing only *Acacia rigidula* on the label – which made up most of the BMPEA-containing products identified by Dr. Cohen and his colleagues. Dr. Cohen said the FDA action was "a day late and a dollar short." I agree.

It is a sad story. The FDA is clearly overwhelmed. Unscrupulous manufacturers introduce two dangerous products for every one the FDA forces off the market. The FDA doesn't act until the products actually kill people, or they are forced to act by public opinion. The bottom line is that we cannot rely on the FDA to keep dangerous products off the market. We need to ignore the enticing claims for effortless weight loss and massive muscle gain from unscrupulous manufacturers. Instead, we should stick with reputable companies with a long track record for manufacturing safe and effective products.

A Bad Week For Sports Nutrition Products

Perhaps the best way to end the section on the danger of some sports nutrition products is to focus on a week in mid-2015 when the chickens came home to roost. It seemed like every time you turned around there was another article about a sports supplement making fraudulent claims, containing illegal ingredients, or harming people. Let me give you just a couple of examples.

Sports Supplements Containing Steroids

Early in the week, the FDA issued a warning to consumers to stop using another sports supplement because of reports of serious liver damage in people using it. The product contained the anabolic steroids methylstenbolone and epistane. There are two important take-home lessons from this incident.

1) The product actually claimed that it contained anabolic steroids. Anabolic steroids are known to cause liver damage, heart attack and stroke, testicular cancer, infertility, and mood disorders. It is hard to imagine why anyone would knowingly use a product that claimed to contain anabolic steroids. Unfortunately, some people are willing to do almost anything that will increase muscle mass and strength.

2) Once again, the FDA often only acted after the product had seriously injured people. I tend to agree with Dr. Cohen that it would be far preferable for the FDA to be proactive and warn consumers about products that have the potential to do harm.

Sports Supplements That Cause Cancer

As if that weren't bad enough, toward the end of the same week a paper[24] was published reporting that the use of muscle-building supplements by young men may increase their risk of testicular cancer by up to 177%. The incidence of testicular germ cell cancer in men 15-39 years old has increased 1.6-fold between 1975 and 2011. The reason for that increase is not known, but the authors of British Journal of Cancer article noted that the use of performance-enhancing supplements in that group has also increased dramatically during the same time period.

A previous study of testicular cancer patients reported that a high percentage of them (~20%) had used performance-enhancing supplements, but no control group was included in that study. Thus, the authors of this study set out to carefully match testicular cancer patients with healthy men of the same age and demographics – something we scientists call a case-control study.

The study compared 356 testicular cancer patients age 18-55 from Connecticut and Massachusetts with 513 controls that were matched by age, race, education, tobacco and alcohol use, exercise level, injury to testes or groin, and family history of testicular cancer. The results were scary.

1) Use of muscle-building supplements increased the risk of testicular cancer by 65% compared to men who never used that kind of supplement.

2) For men who started using muscle-building supplements before they were 25, the risk of developing testicular cancer increased to 121%.

3) For men who used muscle-building supplements for more than 3 years, the risk increased to 156%.

4) For men who used more than 2 types of muscle-building supplements, the risk increased to a whopping 177%. That's almost double.

This study did not identify the actual ingredients that caused the increased testicular cancer risk, but with so many of the muscle-building supplements on the market containing dangerous and/or illegal ingredients it is perhaps not surprising that they might increase cancer risk. After all, this demographic (young males) is the group most likely to choose the "Monster Muscle Builder" products rather the less glamorous, but safer, sports supplements.

I don't want to create the misconception that all sports nutrition products are dangerous. Most are perfectly safe. However, there are a few bad apples in every barrel, and the supplement industry is no different, especially when it comes to sports nutrition products.

Yohimbe: Barking Up The Wrong Tree

I have described the dangers of some sports nutrition products in detail. I could have just as easily talked about dangerous weight loss and energy products. However, let me close this chapter with everyone's favorite sexual enhancement product, yohimbe bark. I recently came across a somewhat disturbing report[25] on supplements containing yohimbe bark published by two scientists at the USDA Agricultural Research headquarters in Beltsville, Maryland.

They analyzed 18 different yohimbe bark dietary supplements for yohimbine, the active ingredient. Of the 18 supplements they analyzed, only one had the amount of yohimbine claimed on the label. Two supplements contained significantly more yohimbine than stated on the label, while the rest contained 0-50% of what was stated on the label. This is particularly disturbing because yohimbine has a very narrow therapeutic index – which is just a fancy way of saying that the difference between an effective dose and a toxic dose is very small.

And yohimbine can be quite toxic! Side effects include gastrointestinal upset and vomiting, anxiety, panic attacks, hallucinations, irregular and rapid heartbeats, high blood pressure, kidney failure, and heart attack. In fact, the FDA has recently classified yohimbe supplements as "potentially unsafe." This classification means that the FDA considers the side effects to be potentially life threatening and is just one step short of an outright ban of the supplement.

What Are The Uses of Yohimbe Bark?

With all this background I was surprised that there were people still selling and using yohimbe bark supplements. So, I decided to go online and research the subject a bit more. I started with PubMed, the National Library of Medicine website for searching peer-reviewed scientific journals. I didn't find any recent articles supporting the efficacy of yohimbe, but I found lots of articles on its toxicity.

One article[26] surveyed Poison Control Centers in 2006 and found that yohimbe supplements accounted for 18% of food and supplement related calls. The only foods generating more calls were the ones containing caffeine because of overuse of all "monster" energy drinks by teens and young adults.

Then I Googled yohimbe. But I skipped over the marketing sites and "muscle madness" sites and went straight to reputable sites like WebMD and the NIH website. It turns out that the only approved use of yohimbine is for erectile dysfunction. It is actually pure yohimbine hydrochloride, not yohimbe bark, that is approved for that use, and it is only available with a prescription. It's also not very widely used for that purpose because it is much less effective than popular brands on the market like Viagra and Cialis.

What Are They Thinking?

Yohimbe bark supplements are still widely used by athletes as a stimulant and to reduce body fat. And they are used by some for their supposed aphrodisiac and hallucinogenic effects. It turns out that the hallucinogenic effects are the only ones that are actually proven. There's no good clinical evidence for the other reported uses of yohimbe-containing supplements.

Interestingly, the USDA study was criticized by an industry spokesperson who said that the study "...was unscientific and betrays a lack of understanding of natural products chemistry." He went on to say "It is established in the scientific literature that there can be a range from 7 to 115 mg yohimbine per gram of yohimbe bark. There is no doubt that the amount of this alkaloid in the yohimbe plant...varies from sample to sample."

I could only shake my head in disbelief. That sounded to me a whole lot more like a reason not to use the yohimbe bark supplements than a reason to use them. My question is: Why anyone would sell – and why would anyone use – a supplement with no proven efficacy, significant risk of toxicity, and with widely varying amounts of the active ingredient from batch to batch?

As I said earlier in this chapter: "What are they thinking?"

Summary: The Good, The Bad and The Ugly

In this section of the book I have focused on the bad players in the supplement market.

1) I have alerted you to products and ingredients that are based solely on hype – for example, products claiming all the benefits of fruits and vegetables in a pill or powder, magical fruits, magical water, methylfolate, methyl B12, and much more.

2) I have shared horror stories of products with no active ingredients, or even worse with toxic ingredients, because of lack of adequate quality controls.

3) I have told you that some product claims are based junk science. The claims sound convincing, but in fact there is no evidence that the products actually work.

4) Finally, I have warned you about products that contain dangerous stimulants, illegal steroids, and other dangerous ingredients. Some of these have actually killed people.

In summary, I have talked about the ugly (products that are dangerous and may even kill you) and the bad (products that are probably harmless, but provide no real benefit). In doing this, I have probably convinced you never to go near a supplement again. Perhaps it is time to talk about the good. There are supplements that actually work – supplements that provide clinically proven benefits. There are also highly ethical companies – companies that:

- Have your best interests at heart.

- Employ stringent quality controls so you know that their products are pure and potent.

- Perform high quality clinical studies that are published in reputable peer-reviewed scientific journals, so you know their products are safe and effective.

Choosing A Supplement Company You Can Trust

I have given you more detailed guidelines for separating the wheat from the chaff at the end of each chapter in this section of the book. Let me close by giving you some simple guidelines to help you choose a trustworthy supplement company.

1) Avoid the hyped claims. If the supplement makes claims like "Get ripped fast," "Intense Energy," "Extreme

Energy," "Eviscerate fat," "Makes fat cells self-destruct," or "boosts testosterone," you should run in the other direction. This alone will help you avoid many of the really bad players in the weight loss, sports supplement, energy, and sexual enhancement markets.

2) Avoid the claims that sound too good to be true. These include things like fruit and vegetables in a pill, magic fruits, magic water, eating chocolate to lose weight and similar claims. If your first thought is "When pigs fly," don't ignore that little voice in your head. It's your common sense speaking.

3) Ignore testimonials. The placebo effect is close to 50% for things like energy and feelings of well-being. In the sports nutrition area if an athlete "thinks" they have more energy every time they work out, they will get stronger – but it will have nothing to do with the supplement they are taking.

4) Ignore endorsements. If even Dr. Oz can be duped, who can you trust?

5) Look for a company that uses rigorous quality control standards in the manufacture of their products. Of course, every company claims they have excellent quality controls, but there are some ways that you can identify the truly good companies.

   o Choose well established companies with a reputation for quality products.

   o Ask them how many quality control studies they do on their products. If it is a single nutrient product, the number should be in the dozens. If it is a multivitamin, the number should be in the hundreds. For more complex products, you should expect a thousand or more quality control tests.

     o   If you are still in doubt, a little research on the internet is sometimes helpful. If the FDA has raised questions about their products or the ingredients in one of their products in the past, I would definitely avoid them.

     o   Finally, sports nutrition products are a special case. In that instance I might recommend that you look for supplements that are used by medal-winning Olympic athletes. Why Olympic athletes? Because Olympic athletes are more rigorously drug tested than any other athlete. They absolutely cannot afford to have any stimulants, steroids or other banned substances in their body at any time. They need products that are pure, safe and effective.

6) Look for published clinical studies showing that the product is safe and effective. Those studies should be done with their product in human subjects, not in cell culture or animals. Those clinical studies should also be published in peer-reviewed scientific journals. If the company just cites their own "studies" or "white papers," ignore them. They may look impressive, but they have not been peer-reviewed. You have no idea whether they are accurate. If you are not familiar with the scientific literature, you might want the see if you can find the article in the National Library of Medicine's PubMed website to be sure that the study was published in a reputable journal. Finally, not every study is well designed. To separate the wheat from the chaff you might want to subscribe to my weekly newsletter: https://health-tipsfromtheprofessor.com.

7) Although I didn't talk about it in this book I also recommend that you avoid products with artificial ingredients. While the risks associated with artificial sweeteners, artificial flavors, artificial colors and artificial

preservatives are not as great as the risks associated with stimulants and steroids, they are still ingredients to be avoided. They provide no real benefits, and we simply do not know the long-term health consequences of artificial ingredients.

I have avoided making specific recommendations in this book because FDA regulations prohibit mixing specific supplement recommendations with the discussions of the effect of supplementation in general at reducing disease risk. Readers of this book can, however, visit my bonus website, https://adesignforhealthyliving.com, for my personal recommendations.

SLAYING THE SUPPLEMENT MYTHS
Section 2: The Myths of the Naysayers

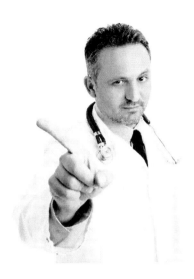

Are supplements going to cure you…or kill you?

Is fish oil good for you…or is it really snake oil?

Are supplements a good investment…or a waste of money?

Do you get all the nutrients you need from food?

I understand your confusion

I have searched the literature to find science-based answers to these questions and more so I can bring you the truth about supplementation

I will guide you through the maze of claims and counter claims so you can choose a supplement program that is best for you.

Introduction

In Section 1 of this book, "The Lies of the Charlatans," I told you about the hype and misleading information you've been given about those "magic" supplements that promise to cure what ails you. I also gave you some practical guidelines on how to separate the hype from the facts.

On the flip side of the coin, you are being told that vitamins don't work. They might cause cancer. They might give you heart attacks. They may even kill you. So, what are you to believe? Where is that truth?

In this section of the book, I'm going to talk about the negative hype – the naysayers and the "myths" about supplementation. But first, let me put this in perspective by reminding you of the "Secrets Only Scientists Know." I covered this topic in detail in my first book, "Slaying The Food Myths." Let me just give you a brief overview here.

1) **We design our studies to disprove generally accepted "truths."** There is no glory to being the 10th person to prove a *paradigm* correct. The glory comes from disproving a paradigm that everybody else thought was true and establishing a new paradigm in the process. Because of this mindset, we are constantly testing and retesting the prevailing paradigms. This is one of the strengths of the scientific method.

2) **Studies often give contradictory results.** In part, this is because they were designed to disprove the scientific consensus. Sometimes we can figure out the reasons behind the differences between study results. Sometimes it's because the study design is different. Sometimes it's because the population groups are different. But quite often, we never really know why one study may say vitamins work, and another study may say they don't. That's why good scientists never base our opinions on a single study. Bloggers, on the other hand, like to quote the studies that support their preconceived notions and ignore the rest. This is something I refer to as "cherry picking" studies to support their hypothesis.

3) **Every clinical study has its flaws.** There is no one perfect clinical study that absolutely proves or disproves a hypothesis. Sometimes it could be the sample size or the sample selection that's flawed. Sometimes it is confounding variables – those unexpected things that influence the outcome. This is one more reason good scientists never accept a single study at face value.

4) **Statistics can be misleading.** Statistical analysis is a very complicated thing, and there are so many ways that it can mislead you. Because of that, we can't just take statistical analyses at face value. We can't just say, "Oh, the statistics prove it." Sometimes we have to ask: "Is that logical?" "What do the other studies say?" "Is there

a confounding variable that they overlooked?" You have to take statistics with a grain of salt.

5) **Scientists are guided by the preponderance of data.** We ask ourselves, "What do most studies on the subject show?" When a new study comes along that contradicts previous studies, we analyze it. If it is an obviously flawed study, we ignore it. If it has no obvious flaws, we designed additional experiments to test it. If those experiments confirm the results of the new study, it becomes the new paradigm. If they refute the new study, it is rejected. Unfortunately, many bloggers don't understand this process. They keep promoting the conclusions of individual studies long after those conclusions have been discredited by subsequent studies.

6) **Scientific consensus takes a long time.** The most obvious example is the original *Framingham Study*. It was in the 50s that we first suspected that high cholesterol was a risk factor for heart disease. But it took another 30 years to prove it so that most scientists believed it was true. That's why good scientists always conclude their papers by saying, "More studies are needed." However, far too many experts have their biases. And when they're reporting to us, they focus only on the studies that support their biases. And the media – bless their hearts – like to hype every single study.

1

Supplement Myths

Now you understand the strengths and weakness of scientific studies. You understand how long it takes to reach consensus in the scientific community. You understand that a single study is almost always flawed. And, hopefully, you understand why a good scientist never accepts a single study – no matter how well designed it appears to be.

With that background in mind, you are ready for a discussion of "supplement myths" and how they arise. In my first book, "Slaying the Food Myths," I talked about how food myths arise. The process is very similar for supplement myths. It starts with a blog or a website. The message is almost always based on the bias of the authors. And, the authors often base their message on misleading information.

- They often confuse animal studies with clinical studies. That's a problem. As I told you in "Slaying The Food Myths," drugs or nutrients that have a particular effect in animal studies only show the same effect in human clinical trials about 10% of the time. So, to cite an animal study and says that it proves a vitamin works or doesn't work – or that it might be dangerous – is not worth a whole lot until someone has actually done the clinical studies to prove that it works in the same way in humans.

- They also tend to quote clinical studies selectively to support their bias. If there are 10 published clinical studies, and they only select the one or two that support their beliefs, you are getting a biased viewpoint. How do you identify the people who are giving you a biased viewpoint? There are lots of them out there. And, most of those people never really let the facts get in the way of a good story. Some of those websites are authored by doctors, but they have their biases, too.

Start by asking whether the message is always spectacular. If their message is almost always spectacular, you know that it can't always be true. If the headlines are usually about miracle foods or nutrients that will prevent Disease X, or about foods and supplements that might kill you, or about things that the establishment isn't telling you, you can probably guess that all their information can't always be true.

Doctors and health organizations also have their biases, and if their bias happens to be anti-supplement, the burden of proof is often applied unequally. That is one of the things that really bothers me as a scientist.

Health organizations and doctors almost always ignore a single study showing benefit. But a single study showing harm is emphasized. Health organizations and doctors immediately warn their patients saying, "You should stop using this," based on a single study. That's not scientific. That's not balanced. That is not based on the weight of evidence.

And then there's the media. As I mentioned above, they have their biases also, and they're not trained in how to interpret scientific studies. They really don't understand about the weight of evidence or how long it takes to reach a consensus.

One of my favorite examples of media bias is a study that was published in 2007 looking at vitamin D and cancer[27]. It was a robust study with almost 17,000 people. The study looked at the effect of vitamin D intake on the 10-year cancer risk.

The results were mixed. There was no effect of vitamin D on overall cancer risk. But, those who were taking in the highest amount of vitamin D were 4-fold less likely to develop colon cancer. So, what did the headlines say? It's kind of humorous. The headlines were all over the map:

- "Vitamin D cuts colon cancer risk"

- "Study finds no connection between Vitamin D and overall cancer deaths"

- "Vitamin D protects against colorectal cancer"

- "Vitamin D may not cut cancer deaths"

- "Scientists advise a Vitamin D downgrade as there is no proof"

Of course, each of the first four headlines was true, but the information in the clinical study was filtered through the biases of the reporters. The last headline was a complete fabrication because the scientists conducting the study really didn't suggest a vitamin D downgrade. So, my question then is, "Who is telling you what to think, and what is their bias?" That's important because they are filtering what they are telling you through their own biases.

More importantly, you have to remember that – whatever the form of media, whether it's online, whether it's TV, whether it's a newspaper – it's the spectacular, the bad news, the things that are different from what everybody else believes that sell subscriptions.

The problem is that once the story has been repeated often enough, it becomes generally accepted as true. It becomes a supplement myth.

B Vitamins and Cancer

Folic Acid and Colon Cancer

Now let's talk about some specific examples of supplement myths. There was a study a few years ago that suggested that 400 IU of folic acid, the RDA for folic acid, increased the risk of colon adenomas in people over 50[28]. Adenomas are benign tumors. They are not colon cancer. But the headlines said, "Folic acid causes colon cancer in people over 50."

Some doctors started recommending their patients only take a multivitamin every other day if they were over 50. For heaven's sake, you wouldn't want to get the RDA of folic acid.

To make matters even more confusing, this single study was picked up by the methylfolate proponents. They claimed it showed folic acid was dangerous, and you should use methylfolate instead. Of course, they were ignoring multiple previous studies that had not indicated any increased risk of either colon adenomas or colon cancer in people taking folic acid. They also ignored the fact that there were zero studies looking at the effect of methylfolate on colon cancer risk. In short, the single experiment suggesting that folic acid might increase the risk of colon cancer was an outlier, and there was no evidence that methylfolate might be any safer than folic acid.

Of course, the study suggesting that folic acid might increase the risk of colon adenomas was followed by a second study. That's what we scientists do. Whenever you have a study that reports something new, other scientists say, "Let's test this. Let's see if we can replicate those results." The second study looked at the effect of 1,000 IU of folic acid, more than twice the RDA, on colon adenomas in people over 50[29]. In that study, there was absolutely no increase seen in adenomas.

But that's not all. That study also asked if you supplement somebody whose folic acid intake was inadequate, were the results different than for somebody who had been consuming adequate folic acid. They found that there was no effect of folic acid on adenomas for the people who had adequate blood folate to begin with. And that makes sense. If you've got enough folic acid in your blood, adding more probably isn't going to make any difference.

However, for those people who had low levels of folate in their blood to begin with, folic acid supplementation reduced adenomas by 40%. That was not an insignificant finding because 55% of the participants in that study had low blood levels of folic acid at the beginning of the study.

Then a third study was performed that looked at 800 IU of folic acid, twice the RDA[30]. This study didn't just measure adenomas. It measured colon cancer, and it showed that 800 IU of folic acid did not increase the risk of colon cancer in people over 50.

Finally, the American Cancer Society decided to do the definitive study[31]. This was a very well-designed study. It measured folates from food and folic acid from supplements, so it measured the total amount of folates and folic acid in the diet from all sources. The study followed 99,523 men and women aged 50-74 for 8 years. And it measured colon cancer – not just adenomas.

This study showed conclusively that high intakes of folic acid, folates, or both did not increase the risk of colon cancer. In fact, it showed the exact opposite. It showed that high intake of folates from food plus folic acid from supplements significantly decreased the risk of colon cancer.

Of course, you hardly saw anything about those studies in the media. They were pretty much ignored because the supplement myth that folic acid causes colon cancer had already been established – even though, by this point, three subsequent studies had disproven it.

Folic Acid And Other Cancers

There have also been a couple of studies suggesting that folic acid might increase the risk of prostate and breast cancer. Some of these were small studies that did not have enough cancer cases to draw a statistically definitive conclusion. Others used mega-doses of folic acid, which I do not recommend. Although these were not definitive studies, they have also been widely hyped by the methylfolate advocates.

Once again, the definitive study appears to have been done[32]. It was a meta-analysis of every placebo-controlled study prior to 2010 that analyzed the effect of folic acid supplementation on cancer risk, a total of 13 studies involving over 50,000 subjects. The results were clear cut. Folic acid supplementation caused no increase in overall cancer risk, and no increase in the risk of colon cancer, prostate cancer, breast cancer, or any other individual cancer. Moreover, the average dose of folic acid in those studies was 2 mg/day, which is 5 times the RDA.

However, the case may not be completely closed for prostate cancer. One recent study[33] reported that while high blood folate showed no association with low grade prostate cancer, it was associated with advanced prostate cancer. This is a single study and requires confirmation. If this finding is confirmed by subsequent studies, it would suggest that while high blood folate does not cause prostate cancer, it may enhance the progression of the disease once someone has prostate cancer. Until we know more, my recommendation would be to avoid mega-doses of either folic acid or methylfolate if you have been diagnosed with prostate cancer.

Vitamins B6 and B12 & Lung Cancer

Another supplement myth is that vitamins B6 and B12 cause lung cancer. You may have heard negative press from the Vitamins and Lifestyle (VITAL) study published in 2017[34]. The headlines in the news said: "Vitamins B6 and B12 Cause Cancer in Men." Once again, the reality was far different than the headlines.

- The increased risk was only seen in men taking mega-doses (more than 20 times the RDA) of B6 or B12 from individual supplements. Multivitamins or B complex supplements containing all the B vitamins in balance did not increase cancer risk. There was also no increased risk of lung cancer for doses of B6 or B12 that were less than 20 times the RDA.

- The increased risk was only seen in smokers. In the words of the authors: "There were too few [lung cancer] patients among never smokers to evaluate associations [between B vitamins and lung cancer]."

The take-home lessons from this study are clear.

- It is almost never a good idea to take mega-doses of individual vitamin and mineral supplements. The only exception is when they are prescribed for a specific condition by your health professional and that health professional is monitoring you for potential toxicity.

- If you smoke, mega-doses of vitamins won't protect you, and they may harm you. The best advice is to stop smoking.

Those are the scientifically based recommendations from the study. However, you are more likely to hear recommendations that you shouldn't take B vitamins if you are a man. After all, supplement myths don't need to be based on science.

Soy and Breast Cancer

Another supplement myth that you've probably heard a lot is about soy and breast cancer. The headlines will tell you that soy consumption increases the risk of breast cancer in women. As with most supplement myths it is based on a kernel of truth that has been blown way out of proportion and has been repeated over and over again long after good clinical studies have proven it to be false.

Let's start at the beginning. The possibility that soy might increase the risk of breast cancer was suggested by studies showing that mice injected with human breast cancer cells and fed soy had an increased risk of breast cancer[35]. Mind you, these were not "garden variety" mice. These were mice that completely lacked an immune system.

There were other animal studies with mice having a normal immune system that came to the exact opposite conclusion[36]. So, the animal studies weren't conclusive. The results were mixed. Yet the headlines blared that "soy may cause breast cancer," and the soy supplement myth was established.

Even if it were true for mice, the important question is whether soy causes breast cancer in women. And the answer to that question appears to be a resounding no! We know from multiple clinical studies that soy consumption over a lifetime decreases the risk of breast cancer by 25-58%[37,38].

What about the effects of soy on breast cancer recurrence in women who have survived breast cancer? Breast cancer survivors have a high risk of breast cancer recurrence, so this is a crucial question. The first clinical study to test the effect of soy on breast cancer recurrence was reported in the December 2009 issue of the Journal of the American Medical Association by researchers at Vanderbilt University and Shanghai Institute of Preventive Medicine[39]. It was a large, well-designed, study that enrolled 5042 Chinese women aged 20 to 75 years old who had been diagnosed with breast cancer and followed them for an average period of 3.9 years.

The results were clear cut. Breast cancer survivors with the highest soy intake had 25% less chance of breast cancer recurrence and 25% less chance of dying from breast cancer than the women with the lowest soy intake. The effect was equally strong for women with estrogen receptor-positive and estrogen receptor-negative cancers, for early stage and late stage breast cancer, and for pre- and post-menopausal women. In short it was a very robust study.

If that were the only published clinical study to test the soy-breast cancer hypothesis, I and other experts would be very cautious about making definitive statements. However, at least four more clinical studies were published shortly thereafter, both in Chinese and American populations. These studies either showed no significant effect of soy on breast cancer recurrence or a protective effect. None of them showed any detrimental effects of soy consumption on breast cancer survivors. A meta-analysis of all 5 studies was published in 2013[40]. This study combined the data from 11,206 breast cancer survivors in the US and China. Those with the highest soy consumption had a 23% decrease in recurrence and a 15% decrease in mortality from breast cancer.

The Soy-Breast Cancer Myth Returns

The soy-breast cancer myth enjoyed a brief revival in 2014 with the publication of a study[41] suggesting that soy might turn on genes thought to influence breast cancer growth. Of course, the bloggers and the media picked this up right away. The headlines screamed: "Soy protein found to speed the growth of breast cancer!" "Eating soy may turn on genes linked to [breast] cancer growth!" "Women with breast cancer should avoid high soy diets!"

Were those headlines justified? Probably not. The authors acknowledged the study had many limitations. For example:

- The increased activity of the cancer growth genes was only seen in 20% of the women studied. For 80% of the women studied, soy protein consumption had no effect on the activity of genes associated with breast cancer growth and survival.

- This effect was only seen for some of the genes associated with breast cancer growth and survival. Other breast cancer growth genes were either not affected or were turned off. The authors conceded that it was unknown whether the genetic changes they observed would have any effect on tumor growth and survival.

- There was no effect of soy consumption on actual tumor growth in any of the women studied.

- The authors acknowledged there was absolutely no way of knowing if the observed changes in gene expression would affect clinical outcomes such as survival, response to chemotherapy, or tumor recurrence.

Several more studies refuting the soy-breast cancer link have been published since 2014, but I should probably touch briefly on a study[42] published in March 2017. That is because the anti-soy bloggers have disputed the validity of previous clinical studies showing the safety of soy by saying most of the studies were performed in China where the amount of soy and type of soy foods consumed are different than in the United States. The 2017 study followed 6235 breast cancer survivors in the San Francisco Bay area and Ontario, Canada for an average of 9.4 years. During that time, 1224 of them died from a recurrence of breast cancer.

- There was a 21% decrease in all-cause mortality for women who had the highest soy consumption compared to those with the lowest soy consumption.

- The protective effect of soy was strongest for those women who had receptor-negative breast cancer. This is significant because receptor-negative breast cancer is associated with poorer survival rates than hormone receptor-positive cases.

- The protective effect was also greatest (35% reduction in all-cause mortality) for women with the highest soy consumption following breast cancer diagnosis. This suggests that soy may play an important role in breast cancer survival.

- The authors concluded, "In this large, ethnically diverse cohort of women with breast cancer [in the US and Canada], higher dietary intake of [soy] was associated with reduced total mortality."

In short, the claim that soy causes breast cancer is just as false in Western societies as it is in China and Japan. It is another example of a supplement myth that doesn't stand up to scrutiny when you look at the studies that have been published since that myth first became popular.

Other Soy Myths

Let me give you a couple of other quick examples of myths about soy that have been disproven. One is that soy interferes with thyroid metabolism. Now, the kernel of truth here is that soy foods can interfere with the absorption of thyroid medication if taken at the same time. That's not peculiar to soy. It's true of almost any food.

But somehow that kernel of truth has been morphed into a warning that if people consume soy protein, they are going to have low thyroid function. There is absolutely no convincing evidence for that. In fact, most clinical studies show that consumption of soy protein has no effect on blood levels of thyroid hormones[43].

The second example is the myth that soy interferes with male fertility. I sometimes joke that somebody forgot to tell that to the Chinese, but that's beside the point. If you look at the clinical studies, they clearly show that soy does not interfere with any measure of male fertility that has been examined[44,45]. These are just more examples of supplement myths that have been disproven but never seem to fade away.

2

More Secrets Only Scientists Know

As a way of introducing the next couple of chapters, let's talk about other secrets that only scientists seem to know. I'll give you a quick overview here, and then discuss each of these examples in depth later.

- One secret that only scientists seem to know is that vitamins aren't magic bullets. They're not drugs. When we talk about nutrition, we really should be focusing on holistic approaches.

For example, we shouldn't be asking whether vitamin C is going to cure anything by itself. Instead, we should be asking whether a diet that is rich with antioxidants and fiber and B vitamins and healthy fats will make a difference. The problem is that 21ˢᵗ century science really is ill-equipped to test holistic approaches. I'm going to go into more detail about this statement in just a minute.

- Another secret that only scientists seem to know is that *primary prevention* is almost impossible to prove. Primary prevention just means that you start with a perfectly healthy population, you give them some intervention, and then you ask down the road: "Does that prevent disease X?"

The problem is that the incidence of disease X in a healthy population is so low that it's almost impossible to prove that your intervention works. I'm going to give you a spectacular example of that in just a minute. However, if you focus on high-risk groups, something called *secondary prevention*, the answer is often different. I'll give you several examples of that as well.

- The other thing to keep in mind is that most diseases take 20-30 years to develop. However, if you do a *double-blind placebo-controlled* clinical trial – the gold standard – 6-12 months is a long time. You are following people under controlled conditions, and you are requiring them to either take your drug or your vitamin or the placebo every single day.

If you're doing *association studies*, where you're comparing populations, 5-7 years is a long time. The bottom line is that many clinical studies are far too short to reliably measure disease outcomes.

- And finally, at the very end of this section of the book, I'm going to give you some examples of what is called *nutrigenomics*. Nutrigenomics is a new frontier, but it's where we really need to go to understand how nutrition is going to affect us as individuals.

3

Holistic Supplementation

Vitamins Are Not Magic Bullets

Let's start the chapter on holistic supplementation by examining the concept that "vitamins are not magic bullets." Once you understand that, you will understand why it's so difficult to show the benefits of individual supplements. The problem is that it's difficult to ask the right questions.

There is the story that I liked to tell every new graduate student in my lab. It goes like this: There is this drunk on the sidewalk, on his hands and knees under a lamppost, just groping around. A policeman comes up to him and says, "What are you doing?" The drunk says, "I'm looking for my house keys." The policeman gets down on his hands and knees, and he looks too. Finally, he says, "I can't find them anywhere. Are you sure you lost them here?" To which the drunk relies, "Nope, I lost them over there, but the light's better here."

The point I try to make by sharing this story is that we can only do experiments where the light is good. But the questions we sometimes want to ask are over in the corner, where we can't really shine the light on them directly. It's difficult to look in the right place – to ask the right questions.

That's particularly the case with holistic approaches because holistic approaches, by their very nature, are multi-factorial. You have multiple variables that you're trying to change at one time. For example, you might want to optimize weight, exercise, vitamins, minerals, and essential fatty acids if you're trying to look at a healthy lifestyle.

But, a 21st century study generally focuses on individual nutrients or individual drugs in an *intervention*, placebo-controlled trial. It's very difficult to evaluate holistic approaches with that kind of study.

The Whole Is Greater Than The Parts

The problem is that the whole is often greater than its parts. One of the examples that I love to use, because it really made an impression on me as a young scientist, occurred at an International Cancer Symposium I attended more than 30 years ago.

I attended a session in which an internally renowned expert was giving his talk on colon cancer. He said, "I can show you, unequivocally, that colon cancer risk is significantly decreased by a lifestyle that includes a high-fiber diet, a low-fat diet, adequate calcium, adequate B vitamins, exercise and weight control. But I can't show you that any one of them, by themselves, is effective."

The question that came to me as I heard him speak was: "What's the message that a responsible scientist or responsible health professional should be giving to their patients or the people that they're advising?" You've heard experts saying: "Don't worry about the fat." "Don't worry about calcium."

"Don't worry about B vitamins." "Don't worry about fiber." "None of them can be shown to decrease the risk of colon cancer."

Is that the message we should be giving people? Or should we really be saying what that doctor said many years ago – that a lifestyle that includes all those things significantly decreases the risk of colon cancer?

Other studies show that holistic approaches are more effective than drugs at controlling Type II diabetes[46]. A holistic approach, something called the DASH diet, is as effective as drugs at controlling hypertension (high blood pressure)[47]. So holistic approaches work, but it's very difficult to prove that individual nutrients or health practices are beneficial. And that's what most of the negative studies that you see in the scientific literature were trying to evaluate.

Holistic Supplementation Versus Individual Nutrients

Here are some examples of the negative press that you may have heard, but where the study actually showed that holistic approaches to supplementation were superior to individual supplements.

There was something called the Iowa Women's Study that got some negative press in 2011[48]. This is one of those studies that led to headlines saying, "Vitamins can kill you." The study did show a slight increase in mortality in people who consumed high-dose individual B vitamins by themselves. But in that same study, people who were taking a high-dose B complex supplement containing all the B vitamins in balance had no increase in mortality. Again, my advice is not to throw away your supplements. Rather you should balance them out and take a holistic approach to supplementation. That's much better than taking high dose individual supplements.

Another example is vitamin E and prostate cancer. You probably saw the headlines, which said: "Vitamin E increases the risk of prostate cancer." Those headlines were based on a study published in the Journal of American Medical Association in 2011[49]. The outcome of this study was puzzling because it contradicted 9 previous clinical trials looking at the effect of vitamin E supplementation on prostate cancer risk. Eight of those studies showed no effect of vitamin E on prostate cancer risk. One study[50] concluded the vitamin E reduced prostate cancer risk.

A follow-up study[51] in 2014 provided an answer to the conundrum. It showed that vitamin E had no effect on prostate cancer risk in men with optimal selenium status. However, it slightly increased cancer risk in men who were deficient in selenium.

There was an editorial[52] evaluation of the paper by some of the top expects in the field that provided thoughtful explanations of the data. The experts pointed out that vitamin E and selenium work together to inactivate free radicals. Vitamin E reduces the free radicals to a chemically unstable intermediate that still has the potential to damage cellular DNA. A selenium-containing enzyme is required to convert that unstable intermediate into a completely harmless compound.

So, when vitamin E is present in much higher levels than selenium, as it was in the group with low baseline selenium status, unstable radicals can accumulate, and DNA damage can occur. The editors felt that this was the most likely explanation for the increased prostate cancer risk when men with low selenium status were supplemented with high-dose vitamin E.

The experts also pointed out that high doses of pure α-tocopherol can interfere with the absorption of the other naturally occurring forms of vitamin E, such as γ-tocopherol – which is the form of vitamin E that decreases prostate cancer risk in animal studies. The experts recommended that you choose vitamin E supplements that contain all the naturally occurring vitamin E forms and contain near RDA amounts of selenium along with the vitamin E.

In other words, the experts were recommending a holistic approach to vitamin E supplementation rather than avoiding vitamin E. These recommendations make much more sense and are a better fit to the data, but don't lend themselves to dramatic headlines – so the editorial has been largely ignored by the press.

The same holistic approach appears to be important if you look at supplementation in general. A study done by Dr. Gladys Block and published in Nutrition Journal in 2007[53] compared people who were taking multiple supplements, typically a multivitamin, extra antioxidants, extra B vitamins, carotenoids, fish oil and probiotics, to people who were taking only a multivitamin, and people who were using no supplements whatsoever over a 20-year period.

The results were dramatic. The holistic supplement users had one-third the prevalence of angina, heart attacks and congestive heart failure and one-quarter the prevalence of diabetes compared to the other two groups. So just like a holistic approach to health, a holistic approach to supplementation appears to be superior.

"Killer Calcium" – Holistic Supplement Design Makes a Difference

One of my favorite examples is the "killer calcium" headlines that came out a few years ago. The headlines said that "Calcium supplements may increase heart attack risk." The original studies suggesting calcium supplementation might increase heart attack risk was published in the British Medical Journal and Heart in the period 2010 to 2012[54,55,56]. But, here's the interesting point. The headlines probably should have said: "Poorly designed calcium supplements may increase heart attack risk."

If you think about most of the calcium supplements in the marketplace, they've been designed based on quick and efficient absorption of calcium into the bloodstream. It's all about how quickly you can get calcium into the blood. If you've been following the hype about calcium supplements over the years, you know that the arguments are all about whether calcium citrate, calcium carbonate, or chelated calcium get into the bloodstream more quickly.

But that's not the question we should be asking. The real question is how effectively that calcium is used for bone formation, something called calcium bioavailability. Because if we just get calcium into the bloodstream and it doesn't go into the bones, it can do some bad things. It gets deposited on the walls of our arteries. That can lead to hardening of the arteries, which could increase heart attack risk. That means if you're just designing the supplement based on how quickly you can get the calcium into the bloodstream instead of how well you can get it into the bones, you might increase heart attack risk.

For efficient bone formation, you also need magnesium and vitamin D. Most, but not all, calcium supplements have those two nutrients. But, you also need things like vitamin K[57], zinc, copper, and manganese for optimal bone formation.

The studies showing the importance of trace minerals in bone formation came from Dr. Paul Saltman's lab a number of years ago. I mention that because it's an interesting and personal story. Dr. Paul Saltman was my wife's research advisor as an undergraduate, and she was involved in some of the research that led to those findings.

In summary, an ideal calcium supplement has more than just calcium alone. It has magnesium, vitamin D, vitamin K, zinc, copper, and manganese. It should be backed by clinical studies showing that it is efficiently incorporated into bone, not just into the bloodstream. Very few calcium supplements meet those criteria. That's why I say that those headlines really should have said: "Poorly designed calcium supplements may increase heart attack risk."

However, I should add a caveat that the headlines linking calcium with heart disease might be inaccurate in the first place. Because the possibility that calcium supplements might increase the risk of cardiovascular disease is a significant health issue, that hypothesis has subsequently been addressed in four major clinical studies[58,59,60,61]. Those studies either found that calcium supplements had no effect on cardiovascular risk or they decreased cardiovascular risk. None of the studies found any evidence for increased cardiovascular risk. For example, the largest of the studies followed 74,245 women in the Nurses' Health Study for an average of 24 years. Here are the results:

- Women taking >1,000 mg of supplemental calcium/day had a 29% decrease in cardiovascular disease and an 18% decrease in cardiovascular deaths.

- When they looked at total calcium intake (dietary and supplemental), women consuming >2,000 mg/day had an 18% decrease in cardiovascular deaths compared to women consuming <500 mg/day (about the average dietary intake for American women).

- It didn't make any difference whether the women were at high or low risk of heart disease (smokers versus non-smokers, high blood pressure versus normal blood pressure, high cholesterol versus normal cholesterol, heart healthy diet or poor diet, pre- or post-menopause).

Once again, we see a familiar pattern. Clinical studies suggest the possibility that supplementation might have an adverse health effect. The bloggers immediate spring into action and another supplement myth is born. Subsequent studies debunk the myth, but the bloggers pay no attention. Supplement myths never die.

Even though the myth about calcium supplements causing heart attacks is probably not true, I still recommend choosing a well-designed calcium supplement. That's likely to be important for strong bones, which is my next topic.

Do Calcium Supplements Reduce The Risk Of Osteoporosis?

On the flip side of the coin, we are also being told that calcium supplements don't increase bone density or reduce the risk of bone fractures. This is also a story about a holistic approach. Before we begin the story, let's start with a little perspective:

The Burden Of Osteoporosis

Osteoporosis is a debilitating and potentially deadly disease associated with aging. It affects 54 million Americans. It can cause severe back pain and bone fractures. 50% of women and 25% of men over 50 will break a bone due to osteoporosis. Hip fractures in the elderly due to osteoporosis are often a death sentence.

For that reason, the RDA for calcium has been set at 1,000 to 1,200 mg/day to reduce the risk of osteoporosis, and calcium supplements are often recommended to reach that target. That's because:

- >99% of adults fail to get the USDA recommended 2.5-3 servings/day of dairy products.

- 67% of women ages 19-50 and 90% of women over 50 fail to meet the RDA recommendations for calcium intake from diet alone.

- Men do a little better (but only because we consume more food). 40% of men ages 19-50 and 80% of men over 50 fail to meet the RDA recommendations for calcium intake from diet alone.

Bone Metabolism And Osteoporosis

Before you can truly understand osteoporosis and how to prevent it, you need to know a bit about bone metabolism. We tend to think of our bones as solid and unchanging, much like the steel girders in an office building. Nothing could be further from the truth. Our bones are dynamic organs that are in a constant change throughout our lives.

Cells called osteoclasts constantly break down old bone (a process called resorption) and cells called osteoblasts replace it with new bone (a process called accretion). Without this constant renewal process our bones would quickly become old and brittle.

When we are young the bone building process exceeds bone resorption and our bones grow in size and density. During most of our adult years, bone resorption and accretion are in balance, so our bone density stays constant. However, as we age bone the bone building process (accretion) slows down and we start to lose bone density. Eventually our bones look like Swiss cheese and break very easily. This is called osteoporosis.

Our Bones As Calcium Reservoirs

We should also think of our bones as calcium reservoirs. We need a relatively constant level of calcium in our bloodstream 24 hours a day for our muscles, brain, and nerves to function properly, but we only get calcium in our diet at discrete intervals. Consequently, when we eat our body tries to store as much calcium as possible in our bones. Between meals, we break down bone material and release the calcium into our bloodstream so that our muscle, brain and nerves can function.

If we lead a "bone healthy" lifestyle, all of this works perfectly. We build strong bones during our growing years, maintain healthy bones during our adult years, and only lose bone density slowly as we age – maybe never experiencing osteoporosis. We always accumulate enough calcium in our bones during meals to provide for the rest of our body's needs between meals.

What is a "bone healthy" lifestyle, you might ask. Because calcium is a major component of bone, the medical and nutrition communities have long focused on calcium as a "magic bullet" that can assure bone health. Once the importance of vitamin D was understood, it was added to the equation. For years we have been told that if we just get enough calcium and vitamin D in our diets, we would build strong bones when we were young, maintain bone density most of our adult years, and lose bone density as slowly as possible as we age. It is this paradigm that the recent studies challenge.

Do Calcium Supplements Prevent Bone Fractures?

Let's look at the studies in question:

- The first study[62] found that achieving the RDA of >1,000 mg/day of calcium increased bone density by an insignificant 0.7-1.8%.

- The second study[63] found that achieving the RDA of >1,000 mg/day of calcium decreased the risk of bone fracture by only 5-10%.

- While the headlines said, "It's better to get your calcium from diet than supplements," the studies actually showed it didn't matter whether you achieved the >1,000 mg/day from diet or supplementation. Neither was effective.

Basically, the authors of these studies concluded that the standard RDA recommendation of 1,000 – 1,200 mg/day of calcium for adults over 50 is unlikely to prevent osteoporosis or reduce the risk of bone fractures.

What Is A Bone Healthy Lifestyle?

There were some significant weaknesses in those studies. However, let's assume for a minute that the studies might just be correct despite their many flaws. Let's assume that the "one size fits all" RDA recommendation of 1,000 – 1,200 mg/day of calcium if you are over 50 may be flawed advice. If so, perhaps it's time to say good riddance! It may finally be time to put away the "magic bullet," "one size fits all" thinking and start seriously considering holistic approaches.

Now that I have your attention, let's talk about what you can do to prevent osteoporosis – and the role that supplementation should play. Let's talk about a "bone healthy" lifestyle.

#1: **Let's start with calcium supplements:** As I said before, bone is not built with calcium alone. Bone contains significant amounts of magnesium along with the trace minerals zinc, copper and manganese – and these are often present at inadequate levels in the diet. Most of us know by now that vitamin D is essential for bone formation, but recent research has shown that vitamin K is also essential. An ideal calcium supplement should contain all those nutrients.

#2: **Next comes diet:** Many of you probably already know that some foods are acid-forming and others are alkaline-forming in our bodies – and that it is best to keep our bodies on the alkaline side. What most of you probably don't know is that calcium is alkaline and that our bones serve as a giant buffer system to help keep our bodies alkaline. Every time we eat acid-forming foods a little bit of bone is dissolved so that calcium can be released into the bloodstream to neutralize the acid. (My apologies to any chemists reading this for my gross simplification of a complex biological system.)

Consequently, if we want strong bones, we should eat less acid-forming foods and more alkaline-forming foods. Among acid-forming foods, sodas are the biggest offenders, but meat, eggs, dairy, and grains are all big offenders as well. Alkaline-forming foods include most fruits and vegetables, peas, beans, lentils, seeds and nuts. In simple terms, the typical American diet is designed to dissolve our bones. Calcium from diet or supplementation may be of little use if our diet is destroying our bones as fast as the calcium tries to rebuild them. Once again, it appears that a primarily plant-based diet is best.

#3: Test your blood 25-hydroxyvitamin D level: 25-hydroxyvitamin D is the active form of vitamin D in our bloodstream. We need a sufficient (20-50 ng/mL) blood level of 25-hydroxyvitamin D to be able to use calcium efficiently for bone formation. We now know that some people who seem to be getting adequate vitamin D from the sun or in their diet still have low 25-hydroxyvitamin D levels. In fact, various studies have shown that somewhere between 20-35% of Americans have insufficient blood levels of 25-hydroxyvitamin D. You should get your blood level tested. If it is low, consult with your health professional on how much vitamin D you need to bring your 25-hydroxyvitamin D into the sufficient range.

#4: Beware of drugs: The list of common medications that dissolve bones is a long one. Some of the worst offenders are anti-inflammatory steroids such as cortisone and prednisone, drugs to treat depression, drugs to treat acid reflux, and excess thyroid hormone. I'm not suggesting that you avoid prescribed medications that are needed to treat a health condition. I would suggest that you ask your doctor or pharmacist (or research online) whether the drugs you are taking adversely affect bone density. If they do, you may want to ask your doctor about alternative approaches, and you should pay a lot more attention to the other aspects of a "bone healthy" lifestyle.

#5: Exercise is perhaps the most important aspect of a bone healthy lifestyle: Whenever our muscles pull on a bone, it stimulates the bone to get stronger. Exercise is so important, I should go into a bit more detail about its role in a bone healthy lifestyle.

The Role Of Exercise In A Bone Healthy Lifestyle

Instead of just quoting more boring studies, I'm going to share a couple of stories that help put the importance of exercise into perspective.

The first is my wife's story. She ate a very healthy alkaline diet with minimal meat and lots of fruits and vegetables for years. She took a very well-designed calcium supplement daily. She walked 5 miles per day and took yoga classes several days each week. She kept her 25-hydroxyvitamin D in the healthy range and took no drugs. Yet when her doctor recommended a bone density scan in her early sixties she discovered she had low bone density. She was in danger of becoming osteoporotic!

Her doctor prescribed Fosamax. My wife tried it for one day and decided the side effects were worse than the disease. So, she started asking holistic health practitioners what she should do. They recommended she find a personal trainer and start pumping iron. That was not an easy solution, but it was the right one. When she went in for her second bone scan 3 months later, her doctor excitedly announced that her bone density had increased by 7%. Her doctor said, "We almost never get results that quickly with Fosamax." When my wife told her she wasn't taking Fosamax, her doctor became even more excited. (Most doctors actually do prefer holistic approaches. They just don't recommend them.)

The moral of my wife's story is that you can be doing everything else right, but if you're not doing weight-bearing exercises – if you're not pumping iron –everything else you are doing may be for naught. Weight-bearing exercise is an essential part of a "bone healthy" lifestyle!

But, can exercise do it alone? Some people seem to think so. That brings up my second story. Over 30 years ago one of my colleagues at UNC, who was an expert on calcium metabolism, was doing a bone density study on female athletes at UNC. One of the tennis players was nicknamed "Tab." Tab was a popular soft drink at that time, and Tab was all she drank – no milk, no water, only Tab. When my colleague measured the bone density of her playing arm, it was normal for a woman of her age. When he measured the bone density of her non-playing arm, it was that of a 65-year-old woman. The reason is simple. When we exercise a particular bone, our body will add calcium to that bone to make it stronger. If we are not getting enough calcium from our diet, our body simply dissolves the bones elsewhere in our body to get the calcium that it needs.

The moral of this story is that exercise alone is not enough. **In terms of bone health, we absolutely need exercise to take advantage of the calcium in our diet, and we absolutely need sufficient calcium in our diet to take advantage of the exercise.**

What About Medications For Preventing Bone Loss?

The danger is that as the studies claiming calcium supplementation doesn't prevent bone fractures get widely publicized and doctors stop prescribing calcium supplements, they probably aren't going to recommend a holistic approach. They won't recommend a "bone healthy" lifestyle. Instead, they will most likely recommend drugs to prevent bone loss.

These drugs have a dark side, and it's not just the acid reflux, esophageal damage and esophageal cancer that you hear about in the TV ads. These drugs all act by blocking bone resorption, the ability of the body to break down bone. In the short term, this prevents the bone loss associated with aging and reduces the risk of bone fractures. However, you might remember from our earlier discussion about bone metabolism that bone resorption is also an essential part of bone remodeling, the process that keeps our bones young and strong. When these drugs are used for more than a few years you end up with bones that are dense, but also old and brittle. Long-term use of these drugs is associated with jaw bones that simply dissolve and bones that easily break during everyday activities.

4

Understanding Clinical Studies

The Three Kinds of Clinical Trials

Now, let's come back to what I said earlier about *primary prevention* versus *secondary prevention*. I made the comment that primary prevention, where you are starting with a healthy population and asking whether your *intervention* can prevent disease X, is almost impossible to prove. To put that into perspective, let me talk about the three kinds of clinical trials.

If you want to determine whether an intervention works, the easiest clinical study is what I call a "treatment study." Treatment studies are what drug companies do. They have designed a drug to treat Disease X. So, everybody in their trial already has Disease X. All they have to do is ask: "Do the symptoms get better?" Or maybe, "Do fewer people die from Disease X?" But everybody in the study has Disease X, so it's relatively easy to prove or disprove whether a drug treatment is going to work.

Secondary prevention is the next easiest way to evaluate an intervention. You are starting with people who are at high risk of Disease X and asking whether you can prevent the disease. For example, you may be starting with people who have already had a heart attack and asking whether you can prevent a second heart attack. If you've got a large enough study population in a secondary prevention trial, you can generally prove whether your intervention will have an effect.

However, primary prevention, as I said before, is very difficult to prove. That's where you're starting with an essentially healthy population, and you're asking, "Can I prevent Disease X in that population?" The problem is that very few people in that healthy population will ever develop Disease X, so it is very difficult to accumulate large enough numbers of people to either prove or disprove whether your intervention will prevent Disease X.

Primary Prevention Studies

Primary Prevention And Sample Size

Sometimes you can overcome that problem simply by increasing sample size. Calcium and colon cancer is a good example of that principle. If you remember what that cancer expert I told you about said 30 years ago, it is very difficult to show that calcium decreases colon cancer risk by itself. For example, there was a study in 2006 with 36,000 women who were given 1,000 mg of calcium carbonate, 400 IU of vitamin D, or a placebo for 7 years[64]. In that study no effect was observed on colon cancer risk.

But that was followed by a very large study a few years later. The NIH and AARP got together. They measured calcium intake from both food and supplements in 500,000 people (that's a lot of people) aged 50-71[65]. They also followed them for 7 years. In that study they were able to show that men who consumed the most calcium, about 1,500 mg a day, had a 20% decrease in colon cancer risk. And women who consumed the most calcium, about 1,900 mg a day, had a 30% decrease in colon cancer. You have to do a very large study to show a benefit when you're looking at primary prevention. Studies that size cost millions of dollars.

Primary Prevention And Statin Drugs

Let me come back to what I think is perhaps the most convincing example of how difficult it is to prove primary prevention. That example is the primary prevention trials with statin drugs. If we look at secondary prevention, statins clearly save lives. If somebody who has had a heart attack is put on statin drugs, their risk of a second heart attack is significantly reduced. But remember, that's secondary prevention. It's a relatively easy thing to prove because a high percentage of the people in that population will suffer a second heart attack in a relatively short period of time. If your intervention reduces heart attack risk, it will be apparent.

However, the drug companies were promoting heavy use of statin drugs in patients who were at risk for heart disease but had never had a heart attack. Some of them were patients with elevated cholesterol, but others were patients who were overweight or had other risk factors for heart disease. It turns out that most of the large drug company-supported trials that had been used to buttress the case for using statins in patients at risk for heart disease had mixed populations. Many of them had already had a heart attack, but some hadn't. The drug companies were promoting statin use for primary prevention of heart disease, but their clinical trials were not pure primary prevention studies.

Because of that, a group of experts came along later and re-analyzed the data. They combined all the studies that the drug companies had done over the years. However, they separated out the subjects who had no previous history of a heart attack or stroke from those who had survived a previous heart attack. In this case they were really focusing on primary prevention. The conclusion from their analysis was that statins could not be shown to reduce the risk of heart attacks in people with no prior history of heart disease[66].

The *Cochrane Systematic Review* published in 2011[67] came to the same conclusion. They also said that you can't show that statins have any effect on the risk of heart attacks in patients who don't have a prior history of heart disease. This is important because the Cochrane Systematic Review is considered the gold standard for evidence-based medicine. They are the people who stringently evaluate all of the existing data and conclude, "This is codified. This works, and this doesn't."

There is an interesting side note here. Cardiologists and the drug companies didn't like that answer, so they asked for a "do-over." The *Cochrane Collaborative* (the group responsible for compiling the Cochrane Systematic Reviews) complied and repeated the analysis, but this time they included studies that had up to 10% patients with prior heart disease. You can think of that as similar to a butcher with his thumb on the scale. That was just enough so that the 2013 Cochrane Review on statin drugs was able to demonstrate a very slight reduction of heart attacks and cardiovascular deaths. The results were more to the drug companies' liking, but this was no longer a pure primary prevention study.

The bottom line is that if you do a true primary prevention trial with statin drugs – which are probably one of the most trusted drugs for reducing the risk of heart attacks – you can't show that they make any difference in preventing a heart attack. Don't misunderstand me. I'm not saying that statins don't work for people who have not yet had a heart attack. I'm just saying that you can't prove that they work in a primary prevention setting.

Vitamin E and Heart Disease Risk In Women

Now that you understand the difference between primary prevention studies and secondary prevention studies and how difficult it is to prove that any intervention makes a difference when you're doing a primary prevention study, let's look at some of the negative statements about supplements that you have heard before.

The Women's Health Study, published in the Journal of the American Medical Association in 2005[68], has gotten a lot of press. That study was done by giving 300 IU of vitamin E or placebo per day for 10 years to 40,000 women – so it was a robust study. And the conclusion, the headline that you've seen over and over again, is that vitamin E could not be shown to reduce the risk of heart attacks or stroke in the overall population.

Of course, now you know that with that population statins probably couldn't have been shown to reduce the risk of heart attacks and stroke either. But you never hear about statins not working. That doesn't fit the bias of the medical profession. You hear about vitamin E not working.

The interesting thing is that in that same study vitamin E reduced cardiovascular deaths by 24%. Somehow, that didn't seem to be worth mentioning. It never made the headlines.

But even more importantly, when they focused on the population over 65, vitamin E reduced the risk of heart attacks and stroke by 25% and cardiovascular deaths by 49%. For women, this is a high-risk group for cardiovascular disease. That's because estrogen protects women from heart attacks, and once they go through menopause their risk of heart attack increases dramatically.

So, when they looked at the subgroup of women in the study who were at high risk of heart disease, the secondary prevention group, vitamin E had some substantial benefits.

That was followed up by the Women's Antioxidant Cardiovascular study in 2007[69]. In this study 8,000 women were given either 600 IU of vitamin E or a placebo every other day. Once again, vitamin E could not be shown to reduce the risk of cardiovascular events in the overall population.

But when they looked at the women who already had cardiovascular disease at the beginning of the study – the secondary prevention group – vitamin E reduced the risk of cardiovascular events by 23%. That is almost exactly the percentage that was reported for the high-risk group in the previous study. So again, in the high-risk groups vitamin E appears to make a difference.

Vitamin E and Heart Disease Risk In Men

Then there is the Health Professionals Study in men[70]. You've probably seen the headlines: "Vitamin E doesn't decrease the risk of heart disease in men." This study is really interesting. This is one where the selection of the study population becomes the deciding factor. But it wasn't because of poor study design. This was self-selection by the men in the study.

The study started with 22,000 male physicians, age 40-84. They were given 400 IU of vitamin E or placebo and followed for 8 years. The study excluded all people who had previous heart attack, stroke, or angina, or who were on blood thinners. So basically, it excluded the high-risk population from the very beginning. But the other interesting thing that happened is another 10,000 of those physicians dropped out because they were unwilling to complete the study.

It turned out that only the healthiest of the healthy – the lowest risk group – were willing to complete the study. When you look at the characteristics of the physicians who self-selected to complete the study, they were 73% less likely to die from heart attack and 67% less likely to die from all causes than the male physician population as a whole.

I think that's probably a "guy thing." We guys just don't want to be part of the study if we're going to look bad. If we already know we're unhealthy, we just say "Why bother? I'm just going to drop out." Only the ones who were really healthy were willing to participate in the study. This self-selection significantly affected the outcome of the study, but it didn't affect the headlines that you saw. That is because the people who write those headlines don't read the papers and evaluate the data. They just look at the conclusions.

B Vitamins – Heart Disease and Cancer

If we look at B vitamins and heart disease, it is a very similar story. There was a primary prevention study looking at supplementation with folic acid, B6 and B12 versus a placebo for 5 years that was published in New England Journal of Medicine in 2006[71]. The headlines that you saw were that B vitamins could not be shown to reduce the risk of heart attacks or death in the overall population.

Supplementation with B vitamins reduced stroke by 25%, but somehow that didn't seem to be worth mentioning. In addition, when they focused on the population that had low blood folate levels at the beginning of the study, B vitamins reduced the risk of heart attacks and cardiovascular deaths by 15%. Simply put, B vitamins decreased the risk of heart attacks in people who had poor diets and were B vitamin deficient.

Another example is a study looking at the effect of supplementation with B vitamins on cancer[72]. This study compared the effects of supplementation with folic acid, vitamin B6 and vitamin B12 versus a placebo for 7 years. The headlines said that B vitamins could not be shown to reduce the risk of breast cancer or total invasive cancer in the overall population. But, when they focused on women over 65, the higher-risk group, the B vitamins reduced the risk of breast cancer by 25% and total invasive cancer by 38%.

So, to sum this all up: If you look at low-risk populations (primary prevention), it's very difficult to show any effect of vitamin E or B vitamins on heart disease or cancer. But remember, the same is true of statins and heart disease risk if you're looking at people at low risk of heart attack. But if you look at high-risk populations (secondary prevention), vitamin E and B vitamins both appear to reduce the risk of heart disease, and B vitamins may reduce the risk of breast cancer.

Secondary Prevention Studies

Vitamin E And Heart Disease

If you look at secondary prevention of heart disease with vitamin E, one of the most famous studies is the Cambridge Heart Antioxidant Study[73]. That study looked at the effect of 800 IU/day of vitamin E or placebo in patients with advanced cardiovascular disease. In that setting, vitamin E significantly reduced the risk of heart attacks and cardiovascular deaths.

Let me be perfectly clear. Not all subsequent studies have agreed with the Cambridge Heart Antioxidant Study. I am not claiming we can say with certainty that vitamin E reduces the risk of heart disease. However, the oft-repeated claim that we know with certainty that vitamin E is ineffective at reducing heart disease risk is equally untenable.

A reasonable interpretation, if you look at all the studies on vitamin E together – if we look at the weight of evidence – would be that if you're at a low risk of heart disease (primary prevention studies), vitamin E can't be shown to reduce your risk of heart attack or stroke. But then, neither can statins. But if you're at high risk (secondary prevention studies), vitamin E may reduce your risk of heart attack, stroke, and cardiovascular death. But if you just read the headlines, you would never know that.

Omega-3 Fatty Acids And Heart Disease

If we look at omega-3 fatty acids, it is a very similar story. The primary prevention studies have been conflicting. However, when we look at the effectiveness of omega-3 fatty acids at reducing heart disease in secondary prevention studies, it is almost like a swinging pendulum. In the 1990s, several strong clinical studies reported that omega-3s reduced heart disease risk. For example, there was the very well-known GISSI-Prevenzione Italian secondary prevention study that looked at the risk of a second heart attack in 11,000 patients from all over Europe who had already had a heart attack[74,75].

That study showed that 1 gram/day of omega-3 fatty acids decreased the risk of fatal attack by 40%. And when they did the statistics, they concluded that with omega-3 fatty acids, 5.7 lives were saved for every 1,000 patients treated per year. That is almost identical to the 5.2 lives saved for every 1,000 patients treated per year with statin drugs.

At that time, everyone was talking about the benefits of omega-3s in reducing heart disease risk. The American Heart Association recommended an intake of 500-1,000 mg/day of omega-3s for heart health. Some experts were recommending even more if you were at high risk of heart disease.

The Pendulum Swings

In the early 2000s the pendulum swung in the other direction. Several clinical studies found no benefit of omega-3s in reducing heart disease risk. For example, a study published in 2012 looked at the effect of omega-3 fatty acids in patients at high risk of heart disease[76]. In this study the participants consumed 1 gram/day of a high purity omega-3 product consisting primarily of EPA and DHA or a placebo. At the end of 6 years no significant difference in heart attack or stroke was observed between the omega-3 group and the placebo group.

As I said previously, when we see two studies that come to very difficult conclusions sometimes we never know why they are different, but sometimes there is an obvious difference. There are two obvious differences between the earlier studies and the 2012 study.

1) In the first place, the criteria for people considered at risk for heart attack and stroke changed dramatically between the 1990s and 2012. Not only has the definition of "high cholesterol" been dramatically lowered, but cardiologists now treat people for heart disease if they have inflammation, elevated triglycerides, elevated blood pressure, diabetes, pre-diabetes or minor arrhythmia.

   For example, the GISSI-Prevenzione study recruited patients who had a heart attack within the past three months, while the 2012 study just looked at people who had diabetes or impaired blood sugar control. While both groups could be considered high risk, the patients in the earlier study were at much higher risk for an imminent heart attack or stroke – thus making it much easier to detect a beneficial effect of omega-3 supplementation.

2) Secondly, the "standard of care" for people considered at risk for heart disease has also changed dramatically. That is important because medical ethics dictates that the control group must receive the standard of care. It would be unethical to withhold a proven treatment from either group. In the earlier studies, patients were generally treated with one or two drugs – generally a beta-blocker and/or drug to lower blood pressure. In the more recent studies, the patients generally received at least 3 to 5 different medications – medications to lower cholesterol, lower blood pressure, lower triglycerides, reduce inflammation, reduce arrhythmia, reduce blood

clotting, and medications to reduce the side effects of the other medications.

Since those medications provide many of the beneficial effects of omega-3 fatty acids, it is perhaps no surprise that it is now more difficult to show any additional benefit of omega-3 fatty acids in patients on multiple medications. However, many experts missed that point. They were now telling us that omega-3s were overrated. They were a waste of money. My favorite headline from that time was "Is Fish Oil Really Snake Oil?" The American Heart Association kept their omega-3 recommendations for heart health, but put more emphasis on omega-3s for people with elevated triglycerides (where the benefits of omega-3s are non-controversial).

Are We Still Asking The Right Question?

The changes in experimental design from the 1990s to the early 2000s meant that we were asking a totally different question. We were no longer asking whether omega-3s reduced the risk of cardiovascular disease in high-risk patients. Instead, we were asking whether omega-3s provided any additional benefit for high-risk patients who were taking 3-5 heart medications, with all their side effects.

However, the people who were writing the headlines were not making that distinction. They were pretending that nothing had changed in the way the studies were designed. They were telling you that the latest studies contradict the earlier studies when, in fact, they were measuring two different things.

I don't know about you, but I'm personally not really interested in knowing whether omega-3 fatty acids or vitamin E are of any additional benefit if I'm already taking three to five medications. I'd like to know whether I can reduce my risk of heart attack and stroke by taking omega-3 fatty acids and/or vitamin E in place of those drugs – as the original studies had suggested.

The Pendulum Swings Back

Suddenly, the pendulum is swinging back again. For example, one recent study[77] enrolled patients suffering from angina or myocardial ischemia and followed them for 10 years. Those with the highest omega-3 status had an 11% decrease in cardiovascular mortality. Another study[78] enrolled patients who just had a heart attack and followed them for 12 months after their hospitalization. All patients received the same care except that one group was prescribed >1,000 mg/day of omega-3s. The omega-3 group had a 35% decrease in occurrence of a second heart attack and a 24% decrease in overall mortality.

Recently, two meta-analyses[79,80] of randomized controlled trials (RCTs) looking at the effect of omega-3s on cardiovascular risk have been published. One meta-analysis included 18 randomized controlled trials with 93,000 subjects. The other included 14 randomized controlled trials with 72,000 subjects. When both meta-analyses looked at patients with no known risk factors for heart disease (primary prevention), omega-3s reduced the risk of cardiovascular death by an insignificant 6-8%. When they looked at patients with one cardiovascular risk factor (either elevated triglycerides or elevated LDL) (secondary prevention), >1,000 mg/day of omega-3s reduced cardiovascular death by 17-18%.

An editorial[81] accompanying one of the articles called the meta-analysis "the most comprehensive of its kind to date…" Those experts went on to say "…omega-3-fatty acid intake of at least 1 gram of EPA + DHA per day, either from seafood or supplementation (as recommended by the American Heart Association) continues to be a reasonable strategy."

As for the American Heart Association, the 2017 Science Advisory from the American Heart Association[82] concluded omega-3 "treatment is reasonable" for secondary prevention of cardiovascular disease and sudden cardiac death among patients with prevalent cardiovascular disease.

As is often the case, you can select one or two studies to support almost any viewpoint about omega-3s and cardiovascular disease. That is what keeps the negative bloggers in business. However, when you look at the preponderance of data (the majority of studies), it is pretty clear that omega-3s reduce the risk of heart attacks and cardiovascular deaths in high-risk populations. In low-risk populations it is reasonable to assume that omega-3s probably reduce the risk of cardiovascular disease, just as we assume (without proof) that statins reduce the risk of heart disease in low-risk populations.

That is an important consideration because many people don't know they are at risk for heart disease until it is too late. For far too many Americans the first indication of heart disease is sudden death from a heart attack or stroke.

Of course, the omega-3 – heart disease controversy will continue. In time, perhaps the most recent studies will come to be accepted by responsible scientists and medical organizations. However, the irresponsible bloggers and anti-supplement groups will probably ignore these studies and continue to tell you that omega-3s are worthless.

5

Problems With Study Design

Multivitamins And Mortality

Let me give you a couple of examples of how problems with study design and statistics have led to inaccurate conclusions. You may have read the headlines saying: "Multivitamins may increase your risk of death." Those headlines were based on an article published in the Archives of Internal Medicine in 2011[83], and they have been repeated so often that this has become one of those negative supplement myths that you hear repeatedly.

That is unfortunate, because this study is an outlier. It is the only study out of dozens of studies on multivitamins that has come to that conclusion. So, the real question becomes why the results of this study differed so radically from all other studies of multivitamins. It was what scientists refer to as an *association study*. It divided the subjects into multivitamin users and non-users, and asked what health outcomes were associated with the two groups.

However, it turns out that the two groups being compared in the study were not balanced. The use of estrogen replacement therapy was twice as prevalent among multivitamin users compared to non-users in this study. That's a very important oversight because estrogen replacement therapy is known to increase the risk of death. In all fairness, the authors tried to control for the difference between the two groups statistically. However, because the outcome of study is so different from all other studies in the literature and it was so heavily biased with the estrogen replacement therapy users, it's hard to be confident that they were able to factor that bias out of the study.

There was one other significant flaw in the study. The authors divided people into multivitamin users and non-users based on their habits at the end of the study. It turns out that the percentage of multivitamin users almost doubled during the study. To make things worse, no effort was made to find out why people who were not taking multivitamins at the beginning of the study started using them.

If you take the time to read all the way to the end of the paper, the authors acknowledged that those people who started using multivitamins during the study may have done so because they started to develop health problems and became more concerned about improving their nutrition. In other words, those people most likely to die may have been the ones who started using multivitamins. Of course, the journalists and bloggers writing the headlines never bother to read all the way to the end of the paper.

The possibility that the sickest subjects started taking multivitamins is a phenomenon that statisticians refer to as "reverse causation," and it has sabotaged many a study. For an example of how reverse causation can give misleading results, see my article on studies claiming eating chocolate aids weight loss in "Slaying the Food Myths." In that article I reported on several studies claiming thin people ate more chocolate than overweight people. Bloggers jumped to the conclusion that chocolate consumption helped you stay slender. Then someone followed a group of people over time and discovered that the people who ate more chocolate gained more weight. In addition, the subjects who developed an obesity-related illness started consuming less chocolate and more fruits and vegetables. Who would have guessed?

And, once again, the positive studies have been ignored. For example, there was a study called the Vitamins Lifestyle Study published in the American Journal of Epidemiology in 2009[84], which followed 77,719 people in Washington state aged 50-76 for 10 years. They compared multivitamin users, vitamin E users, vitamin C users, and non-supplement users. The multivitamin users had a 16% reduction in cardiovascular mortality, and a non-significant reduction in total mortality. Vitamin E users had a 28% reduction in cardiovascular mortality and an 11% reduction in total mortality. Vitamin C users had a 25% reduction in cardiovascular mortality and a 9% reduction in total mortality. That was followed in 2013 by a meta-analysis of 21 studies with over 91,000 people[85]. That study found no association between multivitamin use and mortality.

These results were exactly the opposite of the study that made the headlines. But the positive studies have largely been ignored. It is that unequal reporting of positive and negative studies that create the negative supplementation myths. And, once the myth has been created, it's repeated over and over. It becomes accepted as true, even though the original study is flawed and there are other studies that come to the exact opposite conclusion.

Vitamin E And Mortality

Vitamin E is another example. You may have seen the headlines: "Vitamin E may increase your risk of death." Those headlines came from a single *meta-analysis*, where the authors combined data from a lot of studies and reported that using 400 IU of Vitamin E was associated with a 5% increased risk of dying[86].

Meta-analyses are normally very powerful, but they must be well designed, or their conclusions are meaningless. One problem was that this meta-analysis included only those studies that had adverse outcomes. In other words, if nobody died in a particular clinical study, that study wasn't included. There were hundreds of studies that had no adverse outcomes, and they were completely ignored.

To make matters even worse, the negative results were almost entirely due to a single study in which the vitamin E users were also on hormone replacement therapy. As I mentioned above, we already know that hormone replacement therapy increases your risk of death, so it is suspicious when the only study to show any significant negative outcome with vitamin E was the study in which it was combined with hormone replacement therapy. Once again, the headlines say one thing, but the study design tells you that that conclusion may not be reliable.

Antioxidants And Risk Of Cancer

Another headline you may have seen is that antioxidants may increase your risk of cancer. This study was also a meta-analysis. It combined data from 66 published clinical studies and concluded that consumption of extra vitamins A, E, and beta-carotene were associated with up to a 16% increased risk of cancer[87]. But once again, that study included only those studies in which adverse outcomes were reported. 400 studies with no adverse outcomes were ignored.

More to the point, another group of scientists came back and re-analyzed the same data set a couple of years later[88]. When they looked at same 66 studies included in the original meta-analysis, 60% of the studies showed no effect of supplementation, 36% of studies showed a benefit of supplementation, and only 4% showed an adverse effect. And, once again, that adverse outcome was almost entirely due to the single study in which participants using vitamin E were on hormone replacement therapy.

Since that time, two additional studies have also come to the opposite conclusion. For example:

- One study[89] followed 24,000 adults in Germany for 11 years and found that people consuming antioxidant supplements at the beginning of the study had a 48% decrease in cancer mortality and a 42% decrease in all-cause mortality.

- A US study[90] of 15,000 male physicians found that vitamin C and E supplements had no effect on cancer risk over an 8-year period. But, when the study was extended an additional 3.8 years, vitamin C supplementation decreased colon cancer risk by 46%.

But, of course, these studies have been completely ignored. They didn't fit the convenient biases of the people who really want to hype the danger of supplementation.

Summary: Study Design And Biased Conclusions

So, let me just summarize some things about study design, statistics and biased conclusions:

- Most of the studies that have reported negative or adverse outcomes of supplementation have serious flaws in either study design or statistical analysis.

- Most of the studies reporting negative or adverse outcomes have also been refuted by subsequent studies.

A good scientist would require additional high-quality studies before making any public policy recommendation. But you've seen the headlines. It's those negative studies that make the headlines. They are what become the negative supplementation myths. They are repeated over and over until they become generally accepted as true. The positive studies have largely been ignored.

6

Nutrigenomics – The New Frontier

The Promise of Nutrigenomics

Nutrigenomics is an emerging science I call the "new frontier" of nutrition research. As a Professor at the University of North Carolina I specialized in cancer drug development for over 30 years. Over the last decade a field called *pharmacogenomics*, which is basically looking at an individual's genetic background and how that affects the effectiveness and side effects of cancer drugs, has become widely accepted in the field of cancer drug development.

Because of pharmacogenomics, drugs today are being approved to target cancers for people whose cancer cells have a particular genetic makeup. These drugs would not have been approved a few years ago because if you test them on cancer in the general population, they have little or no effectiveness. They only work on a subset of people who have a form of cancer with a specific genetic makeup.

Nutrigenomics is not far behind. It's the same principle. You've heard for years that we all have unique nutritional needs. Now we are starting to learn why. It's because we all have unique variations in our genetic makeup. The technical term for these gene variations is polymorphisms, but for the sake of simplicity I will refer to them as mutations. These genetic mutations increase our risk of certain diseases, and they increase our needs for certain nutrients.

For example, I have already mentioned that mutations in the *MTHFR* gene increase the risk of certain birth defects, and supplementation with folic acid is particularly important for reducing birth defects in that population group.

Similarly, mutations in the vitamin D receptor, the *VDR* gene, interfere with vitamin D absorption from foods and are associated with a condition known as "vitamin D-resistant rickets". Babies born with this genetic defect require megadoses of vitamin D for normal bone formation. In some instances, they even need to receive 25-hydroxy vitamin D, the activated form of vitamin D.

There are other examples of mutations whose primary effect is to increase disease risk but have the secondary effect of increasing nutritional needs. Let me give you a couple of examples.

One of them has to do with vitamin E and heart disease. This study was called HOPE, the Heart Outcomes Prevention Evaluation study, published in Diabetes in 2004[91]. Like a lot of other studies there was no significant effect of vitamin E on cardiovascular risk in the general population. But there is a particular genetic variation in the haptoglobin gene that influences cardiovascular risk. The haptoglobin 2-2 genotype increases oxidative damage to the arterial wall, which significantly increases the risk of cardiovascular disease. When the authors of this study looked at the effect of vitamin E in people with this genotype, they found that it significantly decreased heart attacks and cardiovascular deaths.

This result was confirmed by a second study specifically designed to look at vitamin E supplementation in that population group[92]. This is another example of a high-risk group benefiting from supplementation, but in this case the high risk is based on genetic variation.

Let's look at soy and heart disease as a final example. There was a study called the ISOHEART study[93,94] that looked at a particular genetic variation in the estrogen receptor which increases inflammation and decreases levels of HDL. As you might expect, this genotype significantly increases cardiovascular risk.

Soy isoflavones significantly decrease inflammation and increase HDL levels in this population group. But they have no effect on inflammation or HDL levels in people with other genotypes affecting the estrogen receptor. So, it turns out that soy has beneficial effects, but only in the population that's at greatest risk of cardiovascular disease. And, this is based on genetic variation.

These are the best-established examples of gene mutations that affect nutritional needs. Many more gene-nutrient interactions have been proposed, but they have not been validated by follow-up experiments.

The situation is similar when we look at gene mutations associated with metabolic responses such as fat and carbohydrate metabolism, obesity, insulin resistance and type 2 diabetes. There are a few gene mutations that have strong associations with obesity and diabetes. Many more gene-metabolism interactions have been proposed, but the data are weak and inconsistent.

Now that you understand what nutrigenomics is and have some background information about it, let's look at the promise of nutrigenomics. One promise of nutrigenomics is personalized supplement programs. We all have different nutritional needs. Wouldn't it be wonderful if someone could analyze your genome and provide you with a personalized supplement program that precisely fits your genetically determined nutritional requirements? There are companies that offer such personalized supplement programs. Are they providing you with something of value or is their testing bogus? Are their supplements worthless?

Another promise of nutrigenomics is personalized diet advice. Some people seem to do better on low-fat diets. Other people do best on low-carb diets. Saturated fats and red meats may be more problematic for some individuals than for others. Wouldn't it be wonderful if someone could analyze your genome and provide you with a personalized diet program – one that allows you to lose weight easily and gain vibrant health. There are companies that will analyze your genome and tell you whether you are more likely to lose weight and be healthier on a low-fat or low-carbohydrate diet. Is their testing accurate or is it bogus? Are they providing you with useful information, or is their diet advice worthless?

The Problem With Nutrigenomics

Now that you understand the promise of nutrigenomics, let's look at some of the problems that have slowed the fulfillment of its promise. The short answer to the questions I posed in the previous section is that personalized supplement and diet programs are on the horizon, but we are not there yet. Companies promising you personalized nutrition programs are misleading you. They quote a few studies supporting the tests they run and ignore the many studies showing their tests are worthless. In case you think that is just my opinion, let me quote from some recent reviews on the current status of nutrigenomics.

For example, a review[95] published in the journal *Nutrients* in 2017 concluded: "The potential applications to nutrition of this invaluable tool were apparent since the genome was mapped. The first articles discussing nutrigenomics and nutrigenetics were published less than a year after the first draft [of the human genome] and an initial analysis of the human DNA sequence was made available...However, fifteen years and hundreds of publications later, the gap between the experimental and epidemiologic evidence and health practice is not yet closed... The [complexity] of the genotype information is not the only factor that complicates this translation into practice; the discovery of other levels of control..., including environment-modulated epigenome and the intestinal microbiome are other complicating factors [I will explain what this sentence means below]... While the science of nutritional genomics continues to demonstrate potential individual responses to nutrition, the complex nature of gene, nutrition and health interactions continues to provide a challenge for healthcare professionals to analyze, interpret and apply to patient recommendations."

Another review[96] published in the journal *Advances in Nutrition* in 2018 concluded: "Overall, the scientific evidence supporting the dissemination of genomic information for nutrigenomic purposes remains sparse. Therefore, additional knowledge needs to be generated..."

In short, the experts are saying we still don't know enough to predict the best diets or the best supplements based on genetic information alone. Why is that? Why is it so complicated? In part, it can be explained by a term called penetrance that I introduced when I was talking about *MTHFR* polymorphisms and the methylfolate myths in Chapter 2 of Section 1 in this book. Penetrance simply means that the same gene mutation can have different effects in different people. In some people, its effects may be barely noticeable. In other people its effects may be debilitating. However, penetrance is just a word. It's a concept. What causes differences in genetic penetrance? Here are the most likely explanations.

1) **Human genetics is very complex.** There are some gene mutations, such as those causing cystic fibrosis and sickle

cell anemia, that can cause a disease by themselves. Most gene mutations, however, simply predispose to a disease or metabolic disturbance and are highly influenced by the activity of other genes. That's because the products of gene expression form intricate regulatory and metabolic networks. When a single gene is mutated, it interacts with many other genes in the network. And, that network is different for each of us. A recent study[97] has estimated that each of us have at least 1,000 unique mutations that affect the activity our genes, 100 mutations that completely inactivate one of our genes and 20 mutations that probably affect disease risk.

2) **Many common diseases are polygenic.** That includes disease like heart disease, diabetes, and most cancers. Simply put, that means that they are not caused by a single gene mutation. They are caused by the cumulative effect of many mutations, each of which has a small effect on disease risk. The same is likely to be true for mutations that influence carbohydrate and fat metabolism and may be true for mutations that affect some nutrient requirements.

3) **The outcome of gene mutations is strongly influenced by our diet, lifestyle, and environment.** For example, a common mutation in the *FTO* gene predisposes to obesity[98]. However, the effect of this mutation on obesity is strongest when it is coupled with inactivity[99] and foods of high caloric density[100] (translation: junk foods and fast foods instead of fresh fruits and vegetables). Simply put, that means most of us are predisposed to obesity if we follow the American lifestyle, but obesity is not inevitable. Data like this go a long way towards explaining the American obesity epidemic.

4) **Epigenetics has an important influence on gene expression.** This is another emerging science I discussed in depth in "Slaying the Food Myths". I will briefly

summarize it here. When I was a graduate student we believed our genetic destiny was solely determined by our DNA sequence. That was still the prevailing viewpoint when the human genome project was initiated. We thought that once we had our complete DNA sequence we would know everything we needed to know about our genetic destiny. How short sighted we were! It turns out that our DNA can be modified in multiple ways. These modifications do not change the DNA sequence, but they can have major effects on gene expression. They can turn genes on or turn them off. More importantly, we have come to learn that these DNA modifications can be influenced by our diet, lifestyle, and exposure to environmental pollutants. This is the science we call *epigenetics*. We have gone from believing we have a genome (DNA sequence) that is invariant and controls our genetic destiny to understanding that we also have an "epigenome" (modifications to our DNA) that is strongly influenced by our diet, lifestyle, and environment and can change day-to-day.

5) **Our microbiome has an important influence on our health and nutritional status.** This is another emerging science I discussed in "Slaying The Food Myths", and I will briefly summarize here. Simply put, the term *microbiome* refers to our intestinal microbes. Our intestinal bacteria are incredibly diverse. Each of us has about 1,000 distinct species of bacteria in our intestines. Current evidence suggests these intestinal bacteria influence our immune system, inflammation and auto-immune diseases, brain function and mood, and our predisposition to weight gain - and this may just be the tip of the iceberg. More importantly, the species of bacteria in our intestines are influenced by our diet. I gave examples of how our diet influences our microbiome and how our microbiome influences our health in "Slaying The Food Myths". However, our

microbiome also influences our nutritional requirements. For example, some species of intestinal bacteria are the major source of biotin and vitamin K2 for all of us and the major source of vitamin B12 for vegans. Intestinal bacteria may also contribute to our supply of folic acid and thiamine. Other intestinal bacteria inactivate and/or remove some vitamins from the intestine for their own use. Thus, the species of bacteria that populate our intestines can influence our nutritional requirements.

Now that you know the complexity of gene interactions you understand why we are not ready to start genotyping people yet. We don't yet know enough to design a simple genetic test to predict our unique nutritional needs. That science is at least 10-20 years in the future, but it is something that's coming.

What the current nutrigenomic studies do tell us is that some people are high-risk because of their genetic makeup, and these are people for whom an optimal diet and/or supplementation is going to make a significant difference. However, because genetic testing is not yet adequate for predicting either disease risk or nutritional needs, most people are completely unaware that they might be at increased risk of disease or have increased nutritional requirements because of their genetic makeup.

7

Who Should Supplement?

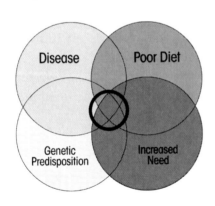

The headlines about supplementation are so confusing. Are supplements useful, or are they a waste of money? Will they cure you, or will they kill you? As usual, the truth lies between the extremes. I feel strongly that responsible supplementation is an integral part of a holistic approach to health. The question is: "Who should supplement and why?"

I created the graphic on the left to answer that question. Now that we are at the end of this book, I can give you specific examples in each of these categories.

Poor diet

You have heard that supplementation fills in the nutritional gaps in our diets. According to the USDA's 2015-2020 Dietary Guidelines for Americans[101], many Americans are consuming inadequate amounts of calcium, magnesium, and vitamins A, D, E and C. Iron is also considered a nutrient of concern for young children and pregnant women. According to a recent study, regular use of a multivitamin is sufficient to eliminate all these deficiencies except for calcium, magnesium and vitamin D[102]. A well-designed calcium, magnesium and vitamin D supplement may be needed to eliminate these deficiencies.

In addition, intake of omega-3 fatty acids from food appears to be inadequate in this country. Recent studies have found that Americans' blood levels of omega-3s are among the lowest in the world and only half of the recommended level for reducing the risk of heart disease[103,104]. Therefore, omega-3 supplementation is often a good idea.

In Chapter 6, I talked about our "microbiome," the bacteria and other microorganisms in our intestine. These intestinal bacteria can affect our tendency to gain weight, our immune system, inflammatory diseases, chronic diseases such as diabetes, cancer, and heart diseases, our mood – the list goes on and on. This is an emerging science. We are learning more every day, but for now it appears our best chances for creating a health-enhancing microbiome are to consume a primarily plant-based diet and take a probiotic supplement.

Finally, diets that eliminate whole food groups create nutritional deficiencies. For example, vegan diets increase the risk of deficiencies in vitamin B12, vitamin D, calcium, iron, zinc and long chain omega-3 fatty acids. A recent study reported that the Paleo diet increased the risk of calcium, magnesium, iodine, thiamin, riboflavin, folate and vitamin D deficiency[105]. The keto diet is even more restrictive and is likely to create additional deficiencies.

Increased Need

We have known for years that pregnancy and lactation increase nutritional requirements. In addition, seniors have increased needs for protein, calcium, vitamin D and vitamin B12. In "Slaying the Food Myths," I shared recent studies showing that protein requirements are increased with exercise.

In addition, common medications also increase our need for specific nutrients. For example, seizure medications can increase your need for vitamin D and calcium. Drugs to treat diabetes and acid reflux can increase your need for vitamin B12. Other drugs increase your need for vitamin B6, folic acid, and vitamin K. Excess alcohol consumption increases your need for thiamin, folic acid, and vitamin B6. These are just a few examples.

More worrisome is the fact that we live in an increasingly polluted world and some of those pollutants may increase our needs for certain nutrients. For example, a recent study reported that exposure to pesticides during pregnancy increases the risk of giving birth to children who will develop autism, and that supplementation with folic acid during pregnancy reduces the effect of pesticides on autism risk[106]. I do wish to acknowledge that this is a developing area of research. This and similar studies require confirmation. It is, however, a reminder that there may be factors beyond our control that have the potential to increase our nutritional needs.

Genetic Predisposition

The effects of genetic variation on nutritional needs is known as nutrigenomics, which I covered in the previous chapter. I gave you several examples of genetic mutations that affect nutritional needs in that chapter. More examples appear in the literature on an almost weekly basis.

Nutrigenomics is an emerging science. We have a lot more to learn. What the existing studies tell us is that some people are high-risk because of their genetic makeup. These are people for whom supplementation is going to make a significant difference. However, because genetic testing is not yet adequate for predicting either disease risk or nutritional needs, most people are completely unaware that they might be at increased risk of disease or have increased nutritional requirements because of their genetic makeup.

Disease

Finally, let's consider the effect of disease on our nutritional needs. If you look at the popular literature, much has been written about the effects of stress on our nutritional needs. In most case, the authors are referring to psychological stress. In fact, psychological stress has relatively minor effects on our nutritional needs. Metabolic stress, on the other hand, has major effects on our nutritional needs. Metabolic stress occurs when our body is struggling to overcome disease, recover from surgery, or recover from trauma. When your body is under metabolic stress, it is important to make sure your nutritional status is optimal.

The effects of surgery and trauma on nutritional needs are well documented. Meeting these needs has become an accepted part of medical practice. However, the effects of disease on nutritional needs is much more controversial. In the earlier chapters, I have discussed the potential effects of disease on nutritional needs in some detail. Let me give you a brief overview here. It is very difficult to show beneficial effects of supplementation in a healthy population (primary prevention). However, when you look at populations that already have a disease, or are at high risk for disease, (secondary prevention), the benefits of supplementation are often evident. For example, studies suggest that vitamin E, B vitamins, and omega-3s each may reduce heart disease risk, but only in high-risk populations. Similarly, B vitamins (folic acid, B6 and B12) may reduce breast cancer risk in high-risk populations. I am not claiming we can say with certainty that supplementation reduces disease risk. However, the oft-repeated claim that we know with certainty that supplementation is ineffective at reducing disease risk is equally untenable. It would be far more accurate to say that supplementation may reduce disease risk in people at high risk for disease, especially if their diet is inadequate.

Who Should Supplement?

With this information in mind, let's return to the question: "Who needs supplements?" Here is my perspective.

1) The need for supplementation is greatest when the circles shown in the figure at the beginning of this chapter overlap, as they do for most Americans. The overlapping circles are drawn that way to make a point. A poor diet doesn't necessarily mean you have to supplement. However, when a poor diet overlaps with increased need, genetic predisposition, or disease, supplementation is likely to be beneficial. The more overlapping circles you have, the more likely you are to benefit from supplementation.

2) The problem is that while most of us are aware that our diets are not what they should be, we are unaware of our increased nutritional needs and/or genetic predisposition. We are also often unaware that we are at high risk of disease. For too many Americans the first indication they have heart disease is sudden death, the first indication of high blood pressure is a stroke, or the first indication of cancer is the diagnosis of stage 3 or 4 cancer.

That is why I recommend that supplementation should be included along with diet, exercise, and weight control as part of a holistic approach to better health.

Summary

At the beginning of this book I said: "Question what you've been told." The myths saying that supplementation does not work or is dangerous are based on:

1) Primary prevention studies, and it is almost impossible to prove that any intervention – even statin drugs – works in a primary prevention setting, or...

2) Studies that suffer from serious flaws in study design or statistical analysis, or...

3) Studies that aren't asking the right question...

In almost every case, the negative studies are balanced by positive studies suggesting benefits from supplementation, especially in a secondary prevention setting. Whenever you identify the populations at the highest risk and with the greatest need, either due to poor diet, existing disease or genetic variations, supplementation appears to be beneficial.

Once again, don't misunderstand me. I'm not saying we have proof that supplementation benefits everyone. As a scientist, I dislike selective use of positive studies to "prove" that supplements work just as much as I dislike selective use of negative studies to "prove" that they don't.

We need more studies. We need more time. Perhaps we need to perfect the science of nutrigenomics before we can assess the benefits and limitations of supplementation for each of us as individuals. My point is simply that claims supplementation is useless or harmful are no more tenable than claims that supplementation offers magical cures. Both are myths.

8

6 Tips For Choosing The Best Multivitamin

As we near the end of this book you have learned about the "smoke and mirrors" many companies use to trick you into thinking they make quality supplements. You have also learned about the scientific basis for choosing a quality product that is both safe and effective. It is time for a practical application of what you have learned. Let me distill that information into 6 tips for evaluating multivitamins. While the tips are specific for multivitamins, the concepts behind them can be applied to almost every supplement. If you learn to use these concepts, you will become good at separating the "wheat from the chaff." You will become a supplement connoisseur.

Let's start with a bit of perspective: There are lots of multivitamin-multimineral products in the marketplace.

Every company must differentiate their product from the competition to win their market share. When that differentiation is based on quality, purity, and clinical proof the product works, I am all for it. May the best company win.

However, the pressure to win market share is intense. Quality controls and clinical studies are expensive. All too often companies try to differentiate their multivitamin-multimineral products based on marketing hype and/or worthless ingredients that subtract money from your wallet without adding anything of value to your health.

With so many claims and counter claims in the marketplace, it has become almost impossible for the average consumer to know which claims are true and which are false. Everyone wants to get the best multivitamin-multimineral for their health at the lowest possible cost. Perhaps that is why I am so frequently asked for guidance on how to choose the best multivitamin. These 6 tips will help you select the multivitamin-multimineral product that is best for you. I will tell you what to look for in a good multivitamin and which marketing claims you should just ignore. Much of what I say has been covered earlier in this book, so I will just summarize briefly here.

Before I give you the 6 tips, I need to review how the nutritional standards for multivitamin-multimineral products are created.

How Are Nutritional Standards Set?

The standards for nutritional supplements are set in a two-step process.

Step 1: In the first step, The Institute of Medicine (IOM) of the National Academies of Sciences selects a committee of experts called the Food and Nutrition Board to set standards for a specific set of nutrients. They set 3 kinds of standards:

- Recommended Dietary Allowances or **RDAs** are the average daily dietary intake levels sufficient to meet the nutrient requirements of nearly all (97-98 percent) healthy individuals in a group.

- Adequate Intakes or **AIs** are established when evidence is insufficient to develop an *RDA* and are set at a level assumed to ensure nutritional adequacy.

- Where toxicity is a potential concern, Tolerable Upper Limits or **ULs** represent the maximum daily intake unlikely to cause adverse health effects.

- Just to confuse things, all three standards are all part of what is called Dietary Reference Intakes or **DRIs**.

Step 2: The DRIs are specific for age, gender, pregnancy and lactation. It would be hopelessly complicated to use DRIs for the nutrition labels on foods and supplements. Therefore, the FDA sets a Daily Value (**DV**) for the purposes of food and supplement labeling. Originally, DVs were set based on the highest DRI for a specific nutrient. However, the FDA has recently devised a new set of DV standards that will be appearing on food and supplement labels starting on July 26, 2018.

Tip #1: Good Product Design Matters

Comparing nutrition labels on multivitamin-multimineral supplements can be tricky. Some supplements only provide 5-10% the Daily Value (DV) for some nutrients. Are those nutrients unimportant? Some supplements provide hundreds or thousands % of the DV for other nutrients. Is more better?

Often companies will quote some random scientist or one or two clinical studies to support the mix of nutrients they include in their multivitamin-multimineral supplement. Don't fall for their marketing hype. The only valid nutritional standards for multivitamin-multimineral products in the United States are set by the Food and Nutrition Board of the Institute of Medicine. They are the standards you should look for in evaluating nutrition labels.

That's because the National Academies of Sciences is the real deal. The National Academies represents the top 1-2% of scientists in the country. To be selected to the National Academies you must be nominated by an Academy member, and voted on by the entire Academy. Selection is based on your research contributions over decades. (No, I am not a member of the Academy, but thanks for thinking that question.)

The Institute of Medicine of the National Academies of Sciences selects the best of the best to serve on the Food and Nutrition Board. They are world renowned experts who review all the pertinent literature (not just one or two studies). They decide on which nutrients are essential and how much of them we need.

It always amazes me that some companies pretend they know more than the Food and Nutrition Board. It amazes me even more that some people believe those companies. With that in mind, this is what to look for when comparing nutrition labels:

- The FDA has set Daily Value (DV) recommendations for 24 vitamins and minerals (23 if the supplement is for adult men or postmenopausal women and does not contain iron). Make sure your multivitamin-multimineral has all 24. Count them. If a company leaves out an essential nutrient, they are not required to list it on the label.

- The Food and Nutrition Board has classified several other nutrients as essential, but does not feel there have been enough studies to establish a DRI. Without a DRI, the FDA cannot set a DV. Those nutrients are represented with a "dagger" symbol on the label with the footnote "Daily Value not established." These are useful additions to a multivitamin-multimineral supplement, provided they are not present in excess.

- Ignore anything companies list on their nutrition labels that does not have a % DV value or a "dagger" symbol. This is often just marketing hype. In some cases, the ingredients have no proven benefit. In many other cases, it's just not possible to put enough of them in a multivitamin-multimineral tablet to provide any real benefit.

Tip #2: Look For Balance

This is another area in which we need to be guided by the recommendations of the Food and Nutrition Board of the IOM. One of the reasons many experts recommend that people get their vitamins and minerals from foods rather than from supplements is because many supplements are unbalanced. That's a problem because there are many cases in which too much of one nutrient can interfere with the absorption or metabolism of related nutrients. For example:

- Zinc and copper compete for absorption. For best absorption and maximal utilization by the body, **the zinc to copper ratio should be close to 1:1 based on DV**.

- B vitamins should be in balance. Look for a multivitamin-multimineral supplement that provides **100-200% of the DV for all 8 essential B vitamins**. (The levels can be higher in a B Complex supplement, but they should still be in balance.)

- Some manufacturers will leave out the expensive B vitamins and load up on the cheap ones. This saves them money. It also allows them to use marketing terms like "mega" or "super." A supplement that provides 50%

or less of the DV for some B vitamins and 1,000% or more of the DV for others is ridiculous. There is absolutely no rationale for a ratio like that except to mislead consumers.

- As for the other nutrients in multivitamin-multimineral supplements, **they should not be significantly below 50% or significantly above 250% of the DV.**

- Unfortunately, the new DVs will introduce some confusion when they start appearing on supplement labels. That's because, in some cases, the new DVs are significantly different than the RDAs established by the Institute of Medicine. I would not fault a company for basing their ingredient amounts on RDA recommendation rather than DVs. However, **there is no good rationale for providing 500% DV or more for any nutrient in a multivitamin-multimineral supplement.**

- Calcium, magnesium, and phosphorous are a special case. They are bulky, so many manufacturers only provide 5-10% of them in their multivitamin-multimineral supplements. This is not ideal because many of the nutrients in a multivitamin-multimineral supplement are required for optimal utilization of calcium and magnesium in bone formation.

- Many Americans get only 50% of the DV for calcium and magnesium in their diet. Thus, it makes good sense to **provide 30-50% of the DV for calcium and magnesium in a multivitamin multimineral supplement.** Most Americans get close to the DV for phosphorous from their diet, so the amount of phosphorous in a supplement is not particularly important.

Tip #3: Ignore The Hype

In their attempts to differentiate themselves, many companies claim that they use a more natural or a better utilized form of the vitamin or mineral than their competitors. Ignore those claims. They are just marketing hype. For example:

- As I covered in Chapter 2, Section 1 of this book, don't believe the claims that methylfolate and methyl B12 (methylcobalamin) are more natural, safer and more effective than folic acid and cyanocobalamin. The claims that alternate chemical forms of other vitamins are more natural, safer, and more effective are equally bogus.

- The claims by some manufacturers that they use a form of calcium that is more readily absorbed is not just misleading, it is the wrong question to ask. Calcium in our bloodstream can do bad things (like calcification and hardening of the arteries) if it is not quickly utilized for bone formation. Thus, the important question is how well the calcium is utilized for bone formation. **Look for clinical studies showing that the calcium in their multivitamin-multimineral supplement is efficiently utilized for bone formation** rather than hype about how quickly it gets into the bloodstream.

- There is a good reason that many supplement companies continue to use traditional ingredients like folic acid for B9, cyanocobalamin for B12, pyridoxine for B6, etc. All of them are supported by hundreds of clinical studies showing that they are safe and effective. As I said previously, there are dozens of studies showing that folic acid supplementation during conception and pregnancy prevents neural tube defects. There are zero studies looking at the effect of methylfolate on neural tube defects. I have no issue with companies choosing to use different forms of these vitamins. Just don't fall for their hype that the forms they are using are some-how more natural, safer or more effective than the traditionally-used forms of the same vitamin.

Tip #4: Don't Fall For Buzzwords

Some manufacturers attempt to differentiate their products by claiming they are natural, organic, non-GMO, or are made from food. The companies are attaching buzzwords to their product that they know resonate with the American people. Don't believe them. Those claims are all bogus. They are mar-keting hype. For example:

- There is no standard for "natural" so companies are not required to provide any evidence to back up their claim. If they claim that their product is natural, **ask for a detailed list of the source and processing method for all their ingredients**. If they are unwilling or unable to provide you with that information, don't believe their claim of natural.

- "Organic" certification for a supplement simply means that ingredients come from crops raised using organic methods. It is no guarantee of purity. Organically grown crops can still be contaminated if the air, soil or water is contaminated from any nearby pollution source. For example, ground water pollution is the major source of the heavy metal contamination often seen in rice-derived ingredients. **It is far more important to select your sup-plement based on rigorous quality control standards that ensure it is pure.**

- **A "non-GMO" designation is useful for foods and for protein, but it is meaningless for the ingredients in a multivitamin-multimineral supplement.** Those ingredients have been extensively purified. They contain no genetic information. They are chemically indistinguishable from purified ingredients obtained from GMO sources. I have no issue with companies choosing to use non-GMO ingredients. It simply represents an unnecessary expense.

- **Claims by some companies that their vitamins are derived entirely from foods are completely bogus. That is a physical impossibility.**

Tip #5: Don't Fall For Scare Tactics

Some companies try to scare you into buying their products by claiming their competitors are using unsafe ingredients. These claims are usually bogus, but it is useful to understand where this misinformation comes from.

There is a lot of unfounded hysteria on the internet about product ingredients. Much of this hysteria has been fueled by a few well-known bloggers. I believe their intentions were pure in the beginning. They started by warning the public about truly dangerous ingredients like artificial colors, flavors, preservatives and sweeteners.

However, blogging has a dark side. To capture a large audience, your blog posts need to be sensational every week. As the weeks go by it becomes harder and harder to find subject matter that is both sensational and accurate. That's when some bloggers go over to "the dark side."

They become more concerned about the size of their audience than the accuracy of the information they post. They start vilifying ingredients that are perfectly safe as long as the manufacturer purifies them correctly and tests them for purity. These are ingredients which might be of concern for products made by a company with poor quality controls, but pose no concern for products made by a company with high quality control standards. In other words, the bloggers should not be spreading hysteria about the ingredient. They should be focusing on some of the real quality control issues in our industry.

Tip #6: Demand Proof

This is the most important tip of all. Many companies make wild claims about their products but feel no need to back up their claims. Ignore their hype and demand they give proof to back up their claims.

- If they claim their products are pure, ask how many quality control tests they run on their products.

- If they claim their products work, ask for proof. Ask for clinical studies:

  o That have been done with people, not with animals, cell culture, or test tubes.*

  o That have been published in peer-reviewed scientific journals.

  o That have been done with their product, not studies done with another product.

*Animal, cell culture and test tube studies are valid if they are used to identify a potential mechanism of action, but should not be cited as proof the product works. For ethical reasons, I prefer companies that do not use animal studies.

The Bottom Line

If you are a regular reader of my "**Health Tips From the Professor**," you know that I end every article with a "Bottom Line" – the take-home lessons from that article. In fact, some of you have told me that "The Bottom Line" is the only part of my articles you read. Here are my bottom line recommendations for supplementation:

- Ignore the hype. There is no convincing proof that supplements cure anything. Supplements are not going to give you effortless weight loss or turn you into an Atlas.

- Ignore the negative myths. There is no convincing evidence that supplements don't work or that they may harm you.

- Your doctors are not trained scientists, and they don't have time to thoroughly analyze the scientific literature. When they give you nutritional advice, they are often just repeating the urban nutrition myths they have heard elsewhere.

- Most of us don't have perfect diets, and supplements can fill the gaps. This is the one generalization that almost every expert agrees with.

- If you do supplement, a holistic approach is best. Avoid high purity, high dose individual vitamins.

- The evidence for the beneficial effects of supplementation is strongest for people who are deficient in one or more nutrients and have increased needs, genetic predisposition and/or are at high risk for disease.

- Unfortunately, most people don't know in advance that they are at high risk for disease. For example, the first symptom of heart disease for many Americans is sudden death.

- Some day we may be able to predict someone's nutritional needs based on their genetic makeup (nutrigenomics), but that day is not now. If someone tries to tell you otherwise, they will probably lie about other things as well.

- Finally, claims that supplementation is useless or harmful are no more tenable than claims that supplementation offers magical cures. Both are myths and should be disregarded.

Free Bonus for Readers of "Slaying the Food Myths" and "Slaying the Supplement Myths": I have covered a lot of ground in these two books. However, I know many of you are wondering: "How does this apply to me? What is the best diet and the best supplementation program for my situation? For that reason, I have put together a personalized guide for healthy eating and supplementation just for the readers of my two books. I call it **"Your Personalized Design for Healthy Living"**, and you can download it for free at my bonus website, https://adesignforhealthyliving.com.

Glossary – Section 1

Arrhythmia: Irregular heartbeat.

Carotenoids: Nutrients found in highly colored fruits and vegetables that are antioxidants and precursors to vitamin A.

Cobalamin: The chemical name for vitamin B12.

Isothiocyanates: Phytonutrients found in cruciferous vegetables that are involved in detoxification of carcinogens by the body.

MTHFR: Methylenetetrahydrofolate reductase is the enzyme responsible for the synthesis of N^5-methyltetrahydrofolate, commonly referred to as methylfolate, in the cell. Related definitions:

- **THF** (tetrahydrofolate) is the most reduced and the biologically active form of folic acid in the cell. There are multiple metabolically active forms of tetrahydrofolate that are generically referred to as folates. However, just to confuse the issue, folate is also sometimes used to refer to both folic acid and the multiple metabolically active forms of tetrahydrofolate.

- **A1298C** is a mutation from A to C at position 1298 of the MTHFR gene.

- **C677T** is a mutation from C to T at position 677 of the MTHFR gene.

- **Homozygote** is two copies of the mutant gene.

- **Heterozygote** is one copy of the mutant gene.

Nutraceutical: A nutraceutical refers to a highly purified nutrient or supplement that provides health benefits in addition to its basic nutritional value.

Penetrance: A genetic term that refers to individual differences in the severity of symptoms associated with a particular mutation. The severity of a given mutation can be influenced by genetic background, diet, and lifestyle.

Phytonutrients: Substances found in plants which are believed to be beneficial to human health and help prevent various diseases.

Thermogenic: To "burn off" calories by increasing the basal metabolic rate.

Tocopherol: The chemical name for vitamin E.

Glossary – Section 2

Cochrane Systematic Reviews: Cochrane Reviews are systematic reviews of primary research in human health care and health policy, and are internationally recognized as the highest standard in evidence-based health care.

The Cochrane Collaboration: The Cochrane Collaborative is an independent nonprofit organization consisting of a group of more than 31,000 volunteers in more than 120 countries. The collaboration was formed to organize medical research information in a systematic way in the interests of evidence-based medicine. The group conducts Cochrane Systematic Reviews of randomized controlled trials of health-care interventions, which it publishes in the Cochrane Library.

Epigenetics: The term epigenetics refers to changes in metabolism or nutritional requirements caused by chemical modification of the DNA or proteins bound to DNA rather than by alterations of the genetic code. These chemical modifications can be influenced by diet, lifestyle, and environment.

Framingham Heart Study: The Framingham Heart Study is a long-term, ongoing cardiovascular study on residents of the town of Framingham, Massachusetts. The study began in 1948 with 5,209 adult subjects from Framingham, and is now on its third generation of participants.

Hormone replacement therapy: Hormone replacement therapy is a form of estrogen treatment used to control menopausal symptoms and in the prevention of osteoporosis.

Hypothesis: A hypothesis is a proposition either asserted as a provisional conjecture to guide investigation (working hypothesis) or accepted as highly probable in the light of established facts.

Microbiome: The term microbiome refers to all the intestinal microorganisms in our body. Our microbiome can be influenced by diet and can, in turn, influence our health and nutritional requirements.

Nutrigenomics: Nutrigenomics is the study of how individual genetic makeup interacts with diet, especially the effects of this interaction on a person's health.

Pharmacogenomics: Pharmacogenomics is the branch of pharmacology that examines the relationships of genetic factors to variations in response to drugs.

Paradigm: A paradigm is a framework containing the basic assumptions, ways of thinking, and methodology that are commonly accepted by members of a scientific community.

Statistical analysis: Statistical analysis is the mathematical body of science that pertains to the collection, analysis, interpretation or explanation, and presentation of data.

Synergistic: When something is synergistic, it means various parts are working together to produce an enhanced result. When synergistic parts work together, they accomplish more than the additive effect of each component acting alone.

Glossary – Section 2
Definitions Related to Clinical Studies

Clinical study: Clinical studies are, by definition, research studies done with humans rather than animals or cell cultures. There are two major kinds of clinical studies, association studies and intervention studies.

Association study (also referred to as a population or epidemiologic study): An association study, is a clinical study that compares health outcomes in populations of people. Ideally, the two population groups are matched in every way except for one variable (vitamin intake, for example) that is being compared. Investigators then ask what health outcomes were associated with the two groups. However, unexpected confounding variables (see definition) can be a problem in this type of study.

Confounding variable: A confounding variable is an extraneous variable whose presence affects the variables being studied so that the results you get do not reflect the actual relationship between the variables under investigation. As an example, suppose that there is a statistical relationship between ice cream consumption and number of drowning deaths for a given period. These two variables have a positive correlation with each other. An evaluator might attempt to explain this correlation by inferring a causal relationship between the two variables (for example, ice cream causes drowning). However, a more likely explanation is that the relationship between ice cream consumption and drowning is spurious and that a third, confounding, variable (the season) influences both variables: during the summer, warmer temperatures lead to increased ice cream consumption as well as more people swimming and thus more drowning deaths.

Intervention study (also referred to as a clinical trial): An intervention study or clinical trial is a carefully designed study that is done with individuals who volunteer to receive an intervention for the treatment or prevention of medical conditions or diseases. In an intervention study, the investigators give the research subjects a particular medicine or other intervention. Usually, they compare the treated subjects to subjects who receive no treatment. Then the researchers measure how the subjects' health changes.

Double-blind, placebo-controlled studies: A double-blind, placebo-controlled study follows a specific set of procedures to ensure that the results obtained are dependable and free from subjective bias. It is considered the 'gold standard' of clinical research studies. Until the study is complete, neither the study researchers nor the participants know who received the study test substance and who received an identical dummy substance, called a placebo. This 'blindness' ensures that the personal beliefs and expectations of either the researchers or the study subjects do not undermine the objectivity of the results.

Primary prevention studies: Primary prevention studies are clinical studies performed in an essentially healthy population to determine whether a specific intervention can reduce the risk of a certain disease.

Secondary prevention studies: Secondary prevention studies are clinical studies performed in a population at high risk of developing a particular disease to determine whether a specific intervention can reduce the risk of developing that disease. An example would be a study performed in group of patients who had survived one heart attack to determine whether an intervention can reduce the risk of a second heart attack.

Meta-analysis: A meta-analysis is a type of research study in which the researcher compiles numerous previously published studies on a particular research question and re-analyzes the results to find the general trend for results across the studies. A meta-analysis can be a useful tool because it can help overcome the problem of small sample sizes in the original studies, and can help identify trends in an area of the research literature that may not be evident by merely reading the published studies.

References

1 J.D. Clarke et al, Pharmacological Research, 64: 456-463, 2011.

2 Patent # US20120315679 A1.

3 C.S. Yang et al, Cancer Prevention Research, 5: 701-705, 2012.

4 J. Mursu et al, Archives of Internal Medicine, 171:1625-1633, 2011.

5 C.H. Hennekens et al, New England Journal of Medicine, 334: 1150-1155, 1996.

6 The Journal of Agricultural Food Chemistry, 56 (3): 627-1158, 2008.

7 B.J. Venn et al, The Journal of Nutrition, 132: 3333-3335, 2002.

[8] I.P. Fohr et al, American Journal of Clinical Nutrition, 75: 275-282, 2002.

[9] P.A. Ashfield-Watt et al, American Journal of Clinical Nutrition, 76: 180-186, 2002.

[10] L.M. De-Regil et al, Cochrane Database Systematic Reviews 2010 Oct 6; (10):CD007950. PMID: 20927767.

[11] J. Durga et al, The Lancet, 369: 208-216, 2007.

[12] A.D. Smith et al, PLoS ONE 5(9): e12244. doi: 10.1371/journal.pone.0012244, 2010.

[13] G. Douaud et al, Proceedings of the National Academies of Sciences, 110: 9523-9528, 2013.

[14] J.A. McMahon et al, New England Journal of Medicine, 354: 2764-2769, 2006.

[15] E. Amster et al, Environmental Health Perspectives, 115: 606-608, 2007.

[16] R.Y. Gordon et al, Archives of Internal Medicine, 170: 1722-1727, 2010.

[17] T.S. Villani et al, Food Chemistry, 170, 271-280, 2015.

[18] J. Bohannon, http://io9.com/i-fooled-millions-into-thinking-chocolate-helps-weight-1707251800).

[19] Z. Harel et al, JAMA Internal Medicine, 173: 926-928, 2013.

[20] A.I. Geller et al, New England Journal of Medicine, 373: 1531-1540, 2015.

[21] D.P. Phillips et al, Journal of General Internal Medicine, 25: 774-779, 2010.

22 P.A. Cohen et al, Drug Testing and Analysis, DOI: 10.1002/dta.1735, 2014.

23 P.A. Cohen et al, Drug Testing and Analysis, DOI: 10.1002/dta.1793, 2015.

24 N. Li et al, British Journal of Cancer, 112: 1247-1250, 2015.

25 M. Condra et al, Journal of Pharmaceutical and Biomedical Analysis, 61: 142-149, 2011.

26 C.A. Haller et al, Journal of Medical Toxicology, 4: 84-92, 2008.

27 D.M. Freedman et al, Journal of the National Cancer Institute, 99: 1594-1602, 2007.

28 B.F. Cole et al, Journal of the American Medical Association, 297: 2351-2359, 2007.

29 J.N. Hathcock et al, American Journal of Clinical Nutrition, 90:1623-1631, 2009.

30 T.M. Gibson et al, American Journal of Clinical Nutrition, 94:1053-1062, 2011.

31 V.L. Stevens et al, Gastroenterology, 141: 98-105, 2011.

32 S.E. Vollset et al, The Lancet, 381: 1029-1036, 2013.

33 A.J. Price et al, European Urology, 70: 941-951, 2016.

34 T.M. Brasky et al, Journal of Clinical Oncology, 35: 3440-3448, 2017.

35 C.D. Allred et al, Cancer Research, 61: 5045-5050, 2001.

36 Z. Jin and R.S. MacDonald, Journal of Nutrition, 132: 3186-3190, 2002.

37 L.A. Corde et al, Cancer Epidemiology Biomarkers & Prevention, 18: 1050-1059, 2009.

[38] B.J. Trock et al, Journal of the National Cancer Institute, 98: 459-471, 2006.

[39] X.O. Shu et al, Journal of the American Medical Association, 302: 2437-2443, 2009.

[40] F. Chi et al, Asian Pacific Journal of Cancer Prevention, 14: 2407-2412, 2013.

[41] M. Shike et al, Journal of the National Cancer Institute, Sep 4 2014, doi: 10.1093/jnci/dju 189.

[42] F.F. Zhang et al, Cancer, 123: 2070-2079. 2017.

[43] B.L. Dillingham et al, Thyroid, 17: 131-137, 2007.

[44] M. Messina, Fertility and Sterility, 93: 2095-2104, 2010.

[45] J.M. Hamilton-Reeves et al, Fertility and Sterility, 94: 997-1007, 2010.

[46] Diabetes Prevention Program Research Group, New England Journal of Medicine, 346: 393-403, 2002.

[47] T.J. Moore et al, Hypertension, 38: 155-158, 2001.

[48] J. Mursu et al, Archives of Internal Medicine, 171:1625-1633, 2011.

[49] E.A. Klein et al, Journal of the American Medical Association, 306: 1549-1556, 2011.

[50] O.P. Heinonen and D. Albanes, New England Journal of Medicine, 330: 1029-1035, 1994.

[51] A.R. Kristal et al, Journal of the National Cancer Institute, DOI: 10.1093/jnci/djt456, 2014.

[52] P.H. Frankel et al, Journal of the National Cancer Institute DOI: 10.1093/jnci/dju005, 2014.

[53] G. Block et al, Nutrition Journal 2007,6:30 doi: 10.1186/1475-2891-6-30.

[54] M.J. Bolland et al, British Medical Journal, 341: c3691, 2010.

[55] M.J. Bolland et al, British Medical Journal, 342: d2040, 2011.

[56] K. Li et al, Heart, 98: 920-925, 2012.

[57] S. Kanellakis et al, Calcified Tissue International, 90: 251-262, 2012.

[58] L. Lansetmo et al, J Clinical Endocrinology and Metabolism, 98: 3010-3018, 2013.

[59] L. Wang et al, American Journal of Cardiovascular Drugs, 12:105-116, 2012.

[60] J.M. Paik et al, Osteoporosis International, 25: 2047-2056, 2014.

[61] L.M. Raffield et al, Nutrition, Metabolism & Cardiovascular Disease, 10: 899-907, 2016.

[62] V. Tai et al, British Medical Journal, BMJ/2015; 351:h4183.

[63] M.J. Boland et al, British Medical Journal, BMJ/2015, 351:h4580.

[64] J. Wactawski-Wende et al, New England Journal of Medicine, 354: 684-689, 2006.

[65] Y. Park et al, Archives of Internal Medicine, 169: 391-401, 2009.

[66] K.K. Ray et al, Archives of Internal Medicine, 170: 1024-1031, 2010.

[67] Cochrane Systematic Review, January 19, 2011.

[68] I.M. Lee et al, Journal of the American Medical Association, 294:56-65, 2005.

69 N.R. Cook et al, Archives of Internal Medicine, 167: 1610-1618, 2007.

70 H.D. Sesso et al, Journal of the American Medical Association, 300: 2123-2133, 2008.

71 The Heart Outcomes Prevention Evaluation (HOPE) Investigators, New England Journal of Medicine, 354: 1567-1577, 2006.

72 N.R. Cook et al, Archives of Internal Medicine, 167: 1610-1618, 2007.

73 N.G. Stephens et al, The Lancet, 347: 781-786, 1996.

74 GISSI-Prevenzione Investigators, The Lancet, 354: 447-455, 1999.

75 R. Marchioli et al, Circulation 105: 1897-1903, 2002.

76 The ORIGIN Trial Investigators, New England Journal of Medicine, 367: 309-318, 2012.

77 M.C. Kleber et al, Atherosclerosis, 252: 175-181, 2016.

78 S.J. Greene et al, American Journal of Cardiology, 117: 340-346, 2016.

79 D.M. Alexander et al, Mayo Clinic Proceedings, 92, 15-29, 2017.

80 K.C. Maki et al, Journal of Clinical Lipidology, 11: 1152-1160, 2017.

81 J.H. O'Keefe et al, Mayo Clinic Proceedings, 92: 1-3, 2017.

82 D.S. Siscovick et al, Circulation. 2017;135:e867-e884.

83 J. Mursu et al, Archives of Internal Medicine, 171: 1625-1633, 2011.

84 G. Pocobelli et al, American Journal of Epidemiology, 170: 472-483, 2009.

[85] H. Macpherson et al, American Journal of Clinical Nutrition, 97: 437-444, 2013.

[86] E.R. Miller et al, Annals of Internal Medicine, 142: 37-46, 2005.

[87] G. Bjelakovic et al, Journal of the American Medical Association, 297: 842-857, 2007.

[88] H.K. Biesalski et al, Nutrients, 2: 929-949, 2010.

[89] K. Li et al, European Journal of Nutrition, 51: 407-413, 2012.

[90] L. Wang et al, American Journal of Clinical Nutrition, 100: 915-923, 2014.

[91] A.P. Levy et al, Diabetes Care, 27: 2767, 2004.

[92] F. Micheletta et al, Arteriosclerosis, Thrombosis and Vascular Biology, 24: 136, 2008.

[93] W.L. Hall et al, American Journal of Clinical Nutrition, 82: 1260-1268, 2005.

[94] W.L. Hall et al, American Journal of Clinical Nutrition, 83: 592-600, 2006.

[95] C. Murgia and M.M. Adamski, Nutrients, 9: 366, 2017.

[96] M. Guassch-Ferre et al, Advances in Nutrition, 9: 128-135, 2018.

[97] D.G. MacArthur et al, Science, 335: 823-828, 2012.

[98] T.M. Frayling et al, Science, 316: 889-894, 2007.

[99] E. Raupersaud et al, Archives of Internal Medicine, 168: 1791-1797, 2009.

[100] J.E. Cecil et al, New England Journal of Medicine, 359: 2258-2566, 2008.

[101] https://health.gov/dietaryguidelines/2015/guidelines/

[102] J.B. Blumberg et al, Nutrients, 9(8): doi: 10.3390/nu9080849, 2017.

[103] K.D. Stark et al, Progress In Lipid Research, 63: 132-152, 2016.

[104] S.V. Thappal et al, Nutrients, 9, 930: doi: 10.3390/nu9090930, 2017.

[105] A. Genomi et al, Nutrients, 8, 314: doi: 10.3390/nu8050314, 2016.

[106] R.J. Schmidt et al, Environmental Health Perspectives, doi: 10.1289/EHP604, 2017.